the teaching voice
second edition

D0870444

the teaching voice
second edition

Stephanie Martin PhD, MRCSLT

Lyn Darnley MSc

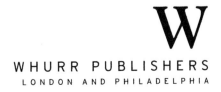

WHURR PUBLISHERS
LONDON AND PHILADELPHIA

MT

© 2004 Whurr Publishers Ltd

First Edition published 1996

Second edition 2004
by Whurr Publishers Ltd
19b Compton Terrace
London N1 2UN England and
325 Chestnut Street, Philadelphia PA 19106 USA

British Library Cataloguing in Publication Data

A catalogue record for this book
is available from the British Library.

ISBN 1 86156 436 8

Typeset by Adrian McLaughlin, a@microguides.net
Printed and bound in the UK by Athenæum Press Limited, Gateshead, Tyne & Wear

3/1/06

Contents

Preface

The first edition of this book was written in response to requests from teachers for information about the theory and practice of the voice, information that many regretted they had not had access to during their professional training.

In this second edition of *The Teaching Voice*, the text has been extensively re-written in response to new developments within the growing field of occupational voice use. Much new research has been undertaken since the first edition was published in 1996 and there continues to be intense interest in the topic, with increasing evidence of the potential for vocal damage as a result of the demands of occupational voice use.

It is hoped that the book addresses a variety of needs, not only to offer detailed information on the subject of occupational voice and the vocal demands of the professional voice user, but also to provide detailed information on the physiology of voice and voice care. Practical advice on aspects of delivery, communication skills and classroom strategies, supported by exercises for developing the resonance, range and projection of the voice, is included.

The book is intended for professional voice users, individuals who use the voice for the purposes of teaching or informing. It aims principally to address the needs of teachers and student teachers in infant, primary and secondary schools, and to be of use to lecturers in the college and university sectors, dance, drama and sports instructors, public speakers in professions such as the clergy and the law, and those in commerce and industry whose professions require communication that is heavily dependent on the voice.

The aim of this book is to offer a mix of practice and theory, which will allow professional voice users to understand how the voice works, to explore some of the factors that influence voice production and, most importantly, to offer readers strategies and solutions that will provide a framework to keep them in good voice throughout their professional career. It is not, however, a substitute for practical teaching which is fundamental to a profession that involves extensive voice use.

This book could not have been completed without the generous support of a number of people. The authors would like to thank them all and to record specific thanks to those within the teaching profession who continue to fulfil such an important role.

About the authors

Stephanie Martin

is a speech and language therapist whose specialist area of interest is occupational voice disorders, with a particular emphasis on the problems experienced by teachers and lecturers. The author of five books, she has completed research projects for the Department of Health and the British Voice Association, and serves as a Council member of the BVA. With a Masters degree in Voice Studies from the Open University, her doctoral research, for which she was awarded a PhD from the University of Greenwich in 2003, explored factors that have an impact on the vocal performance and vocal effectiveness of newly qualified teachers and lecturers. Her professional background includes many years working within speech and language therapy both as a clinician in the UK and overseas, and as a lecturer at University College London, the University of Ulster and the University of Greenwich.

Lyn Darnley

is Head of Voice at the Royal Shakespeare Company. She has teaching qualifications from Trinity College (London), and the University of South Africa and a Masters degree from the University of Birmingham. Her professional background includes working as a performer and voice coach in theatre, television and radio, and in schools, universities and drama schools as a specialist teacher. Before joining the RSC she was Head of Voice at the Rose Bruford College of Speech and Drama. She has maintained contact with drama schools as an external examiner and consultant. Other teaching includes work with universities in Britain and abroad. Other writing includes articles for specialist journals on voice and speech.

The authors' previous joint publications *The Voice Sourcebook* (Speechmark 1992) and *The Teaching Voice* (Whurr 1996) offer a unique perspective on voice as seen from both disciplines.

Acknowledgements

The authors would particularly like to thank:

Lindsay Brown, Rob Day, Mary Johnson, Glyn MacDonald, Shelley Sawers, Heather Steed, Steve Tasker

and the following organisations:

The British Voice Association, The Royal Shakespeare Company, The University of Greenwich

1 The teacher's voice

The teacher as a professional voice user

The generic term 'professional voice user' is often applied to those individuals whose professional role and employment are dependent on effective and efficient use of voice. In the USA, according to Ramig and Verdolini (1998), of a total working population, 24.48 per cent or 28 269 000 individuals had jobs that critically require voice use. In this group may be included, for example, actors, politicians, radio announcers, barristers, the clergy, singers, and teachers and lecturers.

Ascribing the term 'professional voice user' carries with it an implicit expectation that individuals will have had training to bring their vocal skills up to a 'professional' level. It suggests that, by training, expertise and ability, their vocal skills allow them to use their voice effectively in a variety of settings and to different groups and numbers of people. In reality, when teachers are referred to as professional voice users, the term is more accurately describing voice as an essential component of the exercise of their professional role, i.e. the amount of time during their working day that the teacher has to spend talking. In effect, the description refers to the extent of their vocal load, rather than to their competent use of voice or to any previous voice training that has been undertaken.

Jackson (1968) suggests that teachers engage in 200–300 exchanges every hour of their working day, which adds up to 1200–1800 exchanges during their working day, and this does not take into account discussion during breaks or before or after school. In 1993, Masuda et al. analysed speaking behaviour among a group of patients with vocal abuse. When the speaking habits of teachers and patients from other professions who had nodules – small, generally benign, growths – on their vocal folds were examined, it was discovered that these two groups spoke over three times as much as, for example, vocally healthy office workers. The office workers had an average phonation time of 33 minutes over an 8-hour period, whereas the teachers and patients had an average phonation time of 103 minutes over the same period, with half the phonation time at high intensity, or at 80 dB and above. The study also showed that after school phonation time for teachers was very short.

In a recent study of newly qualified teachers and lecturers in their first year in post, Martin (2003) discovered that most respondents reported that they would usually talk for over 60 per cent of each teaching session. This is a considerable amount of time and thus represents high vocal demand and subsequently high vocal loading. In the case of those working within primary education this was consistently at high volume, whereas for those within further education a more balanced use of high and medium volume was reported. If an assumption is made that a similar speech pattern will apply to most teachers, then a picture emerges of extensive speaking periods at high intensity during school and college hours with a much reduced phonation time out of school or college.

Koufman (1998) identifies four levels of vocal usage, which neatly illustrate the link between professional demands and vocal load. Koufman suggests the following categories:

- The Elite Vocal Performer, Level I, is a person for whom even a slight aberration of voice may have dire consequences. Most singers and actors would fall into this group, with the opera singer representing the quintessential Level I performer.
- *The Professional Voice User, Level II*, is a person for whom a moderate vocal problem might prevent adequate job performance. Here, Koufman would include *teachers*, *lecturers* and the clergy (italics are the author's).
- The Non-Vocal Professional, Level III, is categorized as a person for whom a severe vocal problem would prevent adequate job performance. This group includes lawyers, physicians, and businessmen and women.
- The Non-Vocal Professional, Level IV, is a person for whom vocal quality is not a prerequisite for adequate job performance. In this group would be found, for example, labourers and clerks.

Vulnerability of teachers to voice problems

Teachers and lecturers might be surprised to see their professional role featured in such a dominant position on this list, because, for many teachers, any voice work during their training is minimal. Bufton (1997) suggests that, as a result, teachers increasingly form a disproportionately large number of patients attending for voice therapy. A small-scale study in 1992, of 56 speech and language therapy clinics within the UK, recorded an average figure of 6.7 teachers per clinic attending for voice treatment during one specific month (Martin, 1994). In 1997 questionnaires were sent to those same speech and language therapy clinics and the responses obtained from

53 of these clinics showed that the figure had risen to 8.2 teachers per clinic (Bufton, 1997). It was not possible to determine whether this increase was simply a function of general growth, the result of increased awareness of the provision available for teachers with voice problems or an increase in the incidence of voice problems within the teaching population. Morton and Watson (1998) reported that, in a 12-month period in Northern Ireland, 15 per cent of new voice patient referrals were from the teaching profession. As teachers constitute only 2 per cent of the work force in Northern Ireland, this represents a high proportion of the total. In the USA a study of more than 1000 voice patients (Titze et al., 1997) established that teachers constituted 20 per cent of the clinical load. As teachers constitute 4.2 per cent of the workforce in the USA this again seems a disproportionate representation on clinical caseloads.

In other studies in a number of countries, teachers have been identified as a vulnerable group. Questionnaire studies were under taken by Aaltonen (1989) and Pekkarinen and Viljanen (1991) and demonstrated that only 20–30 per cent of the teachers who responded were completely free of any voice problems. More than 10 per cent reported having one or more symptom of vocal fatigue weekly.

A study by Herrington-Hall et al. (1998) explored the occurrence of laryngeal pathologies and their distribution across age, sex and occupation. This study concluded that teaching was one of the top 10 occupations of those who presented with voice disorders, supporting an earlier study by Cooper (1973) where teachers came second in his survey of 956 patients spanning 22 occupations. Several later studies have looked at episodes of vocal attrition among teachers, e.g. Sapir et al. (1993), Martin (1994) and Koufman (1998), and confirm the high incidence of voice problems within this professional group in comparison to other occupations.

A longitudinal study in Brazil (Dragone et al., 1998) followed 69 female elementary school teachers, and compared and contrasted voice quality. A total of 79 per cent of voices were considered to have some degree of alteration after 2 years of teaching; 77 per cent of voices classified as predisposed to voice quality change on the first assessment were considered to have changes in voice quality on the second assessment. Martin (2003) showed that, in a sample of 50 prospective teachers, only 54 per cent presented with a vocal quality, which, on perceptual voice quality rating, was considered to 'be within normal limits'; 30 per cent presented with a vocal quality that was considered to be of slight concern; and 16 per cent presented with a vocal quality that was of definite concern. This predisposing vocal vulnerability was confirmed by the number of those who experienced vocal change during the first term of teaching – all within the sample reported that they experienced vocal change. As a result of the vocal demands of the second term more vocal damage was found to have taken place, which added to the vocal damage sustained in the first term.

Within this study, a different group of teachers and lecturers (number 64), responded to a postal questionnaire sent during their second term in post; half of the respondents reported that they had occasionally lost their voice since starting to teach whereas a sixth had often lost their voice. If these figures were to be generalized to the whole teaching population the numbers affected in the UK would be of great concern.

Occupational health issues

All these studies have demonstrated the effects of teaching on voice problems; certainly the adverse impact on professional careers is well documented. In the UK two groundbreaking court cases within the past 10 years (Oldfield, 1994; Clowry, 1996) highlighted the problems experienced by those in the teaching profession. The courts found in favour of the two teachers whose voice loss, which effectively forced them into early retirement, was agreed to be the result of the demands of their teaching roles.

An ongoing Europe-wide survey on Occupational Safety and Health (OS&H) Arrangements for Voice and Speech Professionals (Vilkman, 2001) recorded responses from 15 countries. Vilkman noted that, using OS&H legislation as a background for the professional voice user, there is a poor level of application of the 1989 Council Directive entitled 'On the introduction of measures to encourage improvements in the safety and health of workers at work'. This directive deals, among others, with such issues as the prevention of occupational risks and the protection of safety and health.

Teacher training provision

Almost five decades ago, West et al. (1957, p. 76) stated:

> No *amount of vigorous vocalization can damage the edges of the vocal folds if the voice is properly used* . . .

Four decades ago Brodnitz (1965, p. 455) wrote:

> *Technically the lack of proper instruction during professional training in the use of the speaking voice is responsible for many voice disorders* . . .

Treatment for vocal abuse and misuse is predicated on the clinical evidence that, for the majority of voice patients, therapy is successful in remediating the problem. Preventive voice care should be successful in mitigating the worst effects of vocal damage and, as a consequence, teachers would be able to monitor and sustain their own voice effectively throughout their working life.

Instructing teachers in voice care can be demonstrated to have a beneficial preventive effect on subsequent vocal damage. A study by Chan (1994) found that a group of 12 kindergarten teachers who explored the concepts and knowledge of vocal abuse and misuse showed voice improvements over 2 months in comparison to a control group. A survey by Martin (1994) revealed that, in a sample of 95 teachers who had received voice training post-qualification, 58 per cent felt that this training session had contributed to a change in their voice and 84 per cent of those who had noted a change stated that this change had been sustained; 77 per cent of respondents had changed their vocal behaviour as a result of the sessions whereas 75 per cent felt that their attitude to their own voice changed as a result of training.

In 1994 Martin highlighted the fact that in the UK few colleges of education offered voice courses for teachers as part of their training. In 1996, the Voice Care Network, in conjunction with the English Speaking Board and the Society of Speech and Drama, published the following resolution:

> *Initial Teacher Education Courses need to provide quality training in use and care of the voice, as the essential tool of professional verbal communication, in order that all intending teachers (both secondary and primary of all subjects) have understanding and practice of how voice is controlled, sustained and adapted for effective verbal delivery that commands respect and gains response.*

In response to the resolution the then chief executive of the Teacher Training Agency (TTA) stated that institutes of teacher training have a duty to ensure that all newly qualified teachers have the necessary skills to communicate effectively in the classroom. Although the TTA does not cover higher or further education, Circulars 9/92 and 14/93, issued to all training institutions by the Department for Education in 1992, stated that, among other things, all qualified teachers must be able to communicate clearly and effectively through questioning, instructing, explaining and feedback (DfE, 1992). This continues to be part of the updated Circulars issued by the Department for Education and Skills (DfES). New standards and requirements included in 'Qualifying to Teach' (TTA, 2002), which apply to all trainee teachers and programmes of initial teacher training from September 2002, state that those awarded qualified teacher status must demonstrate that they can 'communicate sensitively and effectively with parents and carers' (TPU 0803/02-02).

Although the Circular makes no specific reference to voice quality, it could be argued that it should, because vocal quality is accepted as an essential parameter of the communication process (Aronsen, 1985) and vocal attrition compromises the effectiveness of the message. Abnormal voice correlates with negative judgement of personality by children (Lass et al., 1991), so it could be suggested that vocal attrition may adversely affect pupils' perception of their teachers and consequently their education. Evidence shows that a teacher's voice problem can affect pupils' education (Morton and Watson, 1999). In the further education (FE) sector, the Further Education National Training Organisation (FENTO, 1999) proposes a list of 'personal attributes', which are to be displayed by the FE lecturer. These include 'personal impact and presence', attributes in which good communication is implicit but not stated explicitly.

Given these facts it is regrettable that a more consistent and targeted approach to voice care is not yet apparent in teacher training. The General Teaching Council for Scotland is the only teaching council in the UK to have produced a policy document about voice in the teaching profession. The DfES, in their *Healthy Schools, Healthy Teachers* (2001) website, does recommend that teachers and trainee teachers should be referred to specialist help from a speech and language therapist and/or an ear, nose and throat (ENT) consultant should they experience vocal problems.

Suggestions have come from those closely allied to education, e.g. in 1999 Lord Putnam proposed that unemployed actors should give teachers lessons on how to project and protect their voice (Smithers, 1999). Kay Driver, general secretary of the Professional Association of Teachers, addressing the union conference in 1999, said that it was important to convince the government that it was better to try to prevent voice damage than to have teachers off sick and disrupt pupils' education or leaving the professional field (Smithers, 1999).

In 1997 a study investigating the changes occurring between 1992 and 1997 in the provision of voice care education for trainee teachers was undertaken (Bufton, 1997). This study looked specifically at Bachelor of Education (BEd) courses offering students voice care education. In 1992, 36.4 per cent of colleges questioned stated that they made such provision, whereas in 1997 this figure had risen to 45.5 per cent. Although this outcome would initially appear positive, it should be noted that within the same time period the number of colleges where voice care education was compulsory had reduced. In 1992, 87.5 per cent of colleges offering provision stated that students must attend these lectures; by 1997 this figure had reduced to 60 per cent. So, although it may appear that more students were receiving voice care education, in reality fewer may have done so. The survey also raised questions about the number of hours of voice care training to which the students had access, with times ranging from 1 to 18 hours.

One of the most discouraging aspects of the study was the response received to the questions: 'Do you feel that voice care education should be offered on a BEd course?' and 'Do you envisage it being offered as part of the curriculum within the next 5 years?' Only 59 per cent felt that it should be included; others noted that it was important but other issues had to take priority, whereas several institutions stated that time and financial constraints made it impossible to offer students voice care and advice. Few respondents (23 per cent) felt that voice care education would appear on the curriculum within the next 5 years, with the general opinion being that there was neither time nor enough money available. If this was the response from institutions that offered teacher training as part of a 4-year BEd degree it is likely that within a 1-year Postgraduate Certificate in Education (PGCE) time for voice care will be even more limited, with many student teachers from such a course going into schools only 2 weeks after the beginning of the first term.

Vocal requirements for teaching

If teachers are to teach effectively, the undisputed fact is that they need voices that are able to withstand the demands of prolonged voice use often at high volume on a daily basis (Martin, 2003). It is possible to use the voice without tiring, damaging or abusing it for prolonged periods of time, but for all but the most vocally robust this requires prior training – training in how to use and care for the voice effectively and efficiently, and how to manage and monitor the often less than ideal conditions, be these physical or emotional, in which the individual is vocalizing.

Few, if any, teachers work in ideal conditions. Ideal conditions in terms of physical space would be acoustically balanced, warm but not overheated, well-ventilated buildings. Few (if any) teachers are able to produce and sustain vocal quality and volume in an easy and relaxed manner, with well-balanced posture, good control of breath and minimal mental stress over a long period. Factors that contribute to this less than ideal vocal environment are discussed below.

The classroom setting

As has already been noted, the teacher regularly uses his or her voice for a large part of every lesson; recent studies suggest a figure of between 60 and 80 per cent of each lesson as being typical (Ogunleye, 2002; Martin, 2003). Several studies illustrate the fact that noise is a very common and relatively well-recognized vocal health risk factor in teachers' working environments. Noise levels in the classroom place considerable demands on teachers' voices and thereby increase the vocal loading. The Department for Education and Employment upgraded guidelines for environmental design in schools (The Stationery Office, 1997) but before that date there was no information on acceptable noise levels in school classrooms. Smythe and Bamford's study (1997), which looked at speech perception of four primary age hearing-impaired children in mainstream classrooms in the UK, suggests that there should be up-to-date information on classroom acoustics and hearing ability at all levels. They go on to suggest that improving acoustic conditions for hearing-impaired children in mainstream schools benefits the listening conditions for all children and, as a result, has advantages in reduced stress and vocal effort for teachers.

Comins (1995) looked at the difference in noise levels in classes conducted by student teachers and those conducted by experienced teachers, and found a significant difference in noise levels: 66–72 dB(A) for trainee teachers' classes compared with 58–64 dB(A) for the experienced teachers' classes. This study also sought to identify triggers that caused teachers to raise their voices. As the study showed, four of the five trainee teachers raised their voices because the background noise of the children working and talking increased, but this was in effect counterproductive because the pitch of their voices and that of the children's was very close. The male trainee teacher had a lower pitch compared with the children whereas the experienced teacher lowered her pitch instinctively. Although this study was small in scale, it does illustrate the potential for vocal abuse among newly qualified teachers in terms of vocal loading.

Current thinking in education is to encourage children to verbalize ideas and explore language, so that they use speech to explore their world and develop their social and personal skills. Young children are not able, for the most part, to sustain long periods without talking, and indeed anecdotal reports suggest that a similar situation exists in secondary, further and higher education. At all levels within education, group assignments and presentations are increasingly used to examine academic performance. Few would advocate a return to the much more rigid 'silence is golden' philosophy of previous years, but it does, however, create difficulties in terms of voice conservation because there are few periods in the day when the teacher is able to vocalize without competing background noise, be this from pupils, students or indeed computer terminals. It is therefore most important that the teacher develops pedagogical strategies to maximize opportunities for easy voicing.

The teacher or lecturer who has completed a 1-year PGCE course, where classroom practice is fairly concentrated, might be thought to be at more of a disadvantage than those teachers who have been eased gradually into the classroom environment during a 4-year training period; however, there is evidence that vocal loading, the amount of physical load imposed on the vocal folds through movement without recovery time, is particularly critical in terms of vocal abuse and misuse, so that sustained use without rest periods is as important a factor as vocal effort. Teachers, particularly the newly qualified, often find it difficult to assess the degree of vocal effort needed to make themselves heard over a particular level of background noise, and this can lead to early episodes of vocal strain. A recent study (Martin, 2003) found that only 38 per cent of teachers surveyed felt that their voice was equal to the task of teaching.

An unfortunate consequence of vocal strain early on in one's professional life is that, although periods of vocal rest away from school will help to ease the problem (which is why teachers often report that half-term breaks and holiday periods help to alleviate the symptoms), once a pattern has been established it is difficult for the teacher to alter his or her method of talking without help. Help from an outside agency once the teacher begins to work and to experience difficulties may be difficult to access or arrange, which is why training before the teacher goes into the classroom is so essential. Chapters 8–10 explore strategies, and Chapters 11 and 12 offer practical exercises, for dealing with many of the vocally demanding aspects of teaching.

Classroom design

Even when background noise is not a problem, classroom design is often ill thought out in terms of the demands that it places on the teacher's voice. Hargreaves (1984), commenting on the constraints placed on teaching activity 20 years ago, cites material constraints such as school buildings, resources and class size. Although his considerations are not of the significant effect of these constraints on the teacher's voice, it is interesting to note his comments:

> . . . *as a result, teachers now work within widely variant architectural constraints; some in old 1870 buildings and others who are fortunate enough to be working in areas of expanding population in modern open-plan units.*
>
> Hargreaves, 1984 (p. 69)

Although acknowledging his comment that modern open-plan units may be favoured by teachers, there is, in fact, little to choose between them and older schools in terms of their acoustic profile and the vocal problems that they present. New schools are built to encourage openness, which is invaluable in terms of the school functioning as a community, but it is much more difficult to use the voice effectively in large open spaces. The structure of buildings and the materials used inside them determine their ultimate acoustic quality. In general, low ceilings, carpeted floors, covered walls and soft furnishings tend to 'dampen and deaden' sound and consequently absorb the voice. Hard surfaces, such as varnished timber or wooden tiles, steel-framed windows and doors, large expanses of glass and bare walls, tend to produce a bright, sharp and occasionally echoing sound.

Borrild (1978) defines a good acoustic environment as providing conditions in which noise is suppressed and useful sounds stand out clearly and are easily distinguishable. Working in new purpose-built, high-tech schools with lots of glass, exposed brickwork and open spaces is often just as demanding vocally as working in older schools. Older schools, which range from those housed in their original nineteenth century buildings with cathedral roofs to the glass and concrete structures of the 1960s so beloved of new town planners, all have their own problems acoustically and environmentally, and these should not be overlooked. The effect on the voice of the acoustic space is very important to the teacher. Primary school teachers often spend their whole day teaching in one space; teachers and lecturers in the secondary and tertiary sectors find that they have to work in a variety of spaces. It is encouraging to note an increased awareness within education of the importance of the teaching environment. Regulations about spatial requirements and the acoustic property of the teaching space are receiving increased attention at all levels.

Classrooms are principally arranged to accommodate the needs of the pupils, rather than providing for the vocal needs of the teacher. Teachers and lecturers working in large spaces such as lecture rooms and large classrooms encounter problems related to the natural loss of sound over distance, e.g. at a distance of 6 m, sounds are only a quarter as strong as they were at a distance of 3 m. At 12 m they are only a little over a twentieth as strong as they were at 3 m. For many teachers and lecturers, the problems of teaching a class in a large space is one of attempting to 'reach' those at the back without too much vocal effort. Martin (2003) reports that 41 per cent of teachers sampled admitted that they occasionally had difficulty making themselves heard in class. If teachers are unable to modify their teaching voice to accommodate the acoustics of the space, then they will, for the most part, be attempting to counteract the effect by potentially vocally abusive behaviours such as pushing or straining the voice or increasing the volume.

In infant and primary classes children sit on small chairs around small tables – a seating plan that is designed to encourage conversation and to give the small child security and a feeling of being at home in a friendly environment. This is obviously important in terms of creating a positive learning environment, but it does offer unlimited opportunities for the children to talk among themselves, thus increasing the level of background noise over which the teacher has to speak. It also places increased strain on the vocal mechanism because the height of the tables means that the teacher, in order to make eye contact when talking to the pupils, has either to crouch by the side of the table or to bend over. Later chapters

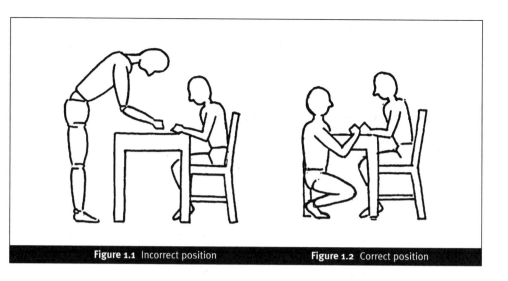

Figure 1.1 Incorrect position   **Figure 1.2** Correct position

give more information on the anatomy and structure of the larynx and how the voice is affected both directly and indirectly by postural changes, but it is important to stress, at this point, that bending awkwardly and vocalizing at the same time is not conducive to easy voicing. Crouching, although possibly less dignified, is more vocally desirable because it maintains the important head/neck alignment and thus prevents strain on the external and internal musculature of the larynx. Crouching or bending at the knee requires much more conscious effort on the part of the teacher, who on spontaneously responding to a pupil will instinctively tend to bend rather than to crouch, with concomitant strain on the back, neck and ultimately the voice.

Actors who are required to perform in physically limiting positions would generally insist on being taught the necessary physical and vocal techniques in order to prevent vocal strain, if necessary involving the support of their union. It is regrettable that the same does not apply to the teaching profession, where there has been limited recognition of the vocal demands of teaching and a gross underestimation of the need to train the teacher's voice. Commerce, industry and politics acknowledge the benefit of training in voice and communication skills, so why has the teacher been overlooked for so long?

One reason may be that, within the teaching profession, there appears to be a tacit acceptance that voice problems 'come with the territory': if you teach you expect to have voice problems. The received wisdom seems to be that these will occur with more or less frequency and be of greater or lesser severity according to 'luck'. You are lucky if you get through a term without a problem. In fact there is no scientific proof that luck plays any part in the maintenance of good voice, but what is undisputed is the fact that voice care and development training could greatly enhance the ability of teachers to sustain voice with little effort, during prolonged periods of teaching.

Additional factors affecting voice

In assessing the vocal demands of the teaching role, the extra, vocally demanding duties that teachers undertake are often forgotten. Responsibilities such as playground duty mean that many teachers end up shouting to gain attention out of doors in all weather. Similarly with sports activities, where children are generally noisy and very excited, teachers often have no other recourse than to shout when trying to gain their attention. Shouting under stress, unless done properly through a learned technique, is potentially very vocally abusive.

Sports classes held inside in a gym with little ventilation are also full of vocal 'minefields', but possibly the most difficult situation of all is where a teacher has to supervise pupils in echoing swimming pools. One teacher remarked that her voice had never been the same since she started to teach groups of pupils swimming at a municipal baths. She simply tried to shout louder to make herself heard and ended up experiencing quite severe vocal strain.

Although there is an acceptance that certain extracurricular activities do require special skills and allowances are given, there are very few occasions on which recommendations are made regarding the vocal skills required. Drama classes, music and singing classes form part of the primary teacher's role and indeed music is an essential component of teaching within the primary school. For many teachers, these vocally demanding activities prove to be too much and their voices 'break down', sometimes resulting in the need to change profession. Anecdotal reports from teachers confirm, for example, that they used to be able to sing but now cannot do more than guide and monitor their pupils – their vocal range has dramatically diminished. That is not to suggest that these activities should be omitted, but rather to recognize that many teachers who have acquired skills in an ad hoc manner, as a result of their teaching experience, need additional training to cope with such intense vocal demands.

Many teachers feel pressured to undertake after-school clubs, activities and sporting fixtures. One junior school, known to the authors, has 35 after-school activities on offer to pupils and this school is not an exception. Not to be seen to play a full and active part in the school by 'volunteering' for these extracurricular activities may be seen as tantamount to signalling that you are not willing to give your full support to the school, or that you have limited interest in promotion or advancement within the profession.

Repetitive strain injury (RSI) has enjoyed considerable attention worldwide, and indeed has been proved to be a painful and distressing side effect for many workers. Substantial damages have been awarded to those who had suffered RSI and could prove that this had occurred as a function of their working life. Increased attention has now been focused on what could be described as 'RSI of the vocal folds' in terms of occupational voice disorders. What researchers are investigating is the link between the strain imposed on the vocal folds through sustained voicing over long periods and the amount of recovery time that is available to the individual. Emerging evidence from call centre personnel shows that many are experiencing significant vocal problems as a result of the unremitting vocal output with limited recovery time – showing vocal changes very similar to those experienced and reported over decades by teachers and lecturers.

Voice care

Earlier in this chapter aspects of training provision were highlighted as was the increased concern shown by the European Union for issues of occupational health. Although this attention is welcome it would also be encouraging to note more direct involvement by the teaching profession to give voice care and development a higher priority. Martin (1994, 2003) showed that, although those teachers interviewed regarded their voice as an important professional tool, 92 per cent reported that fellow staff members did not see voice care as important.

Yet, alongside the wastage to the profession from those whose voice problems prevent them from continuing in their professional role should be set the many hundreds of hours lost through laryngitis, episodic voice loss and vocal abuse experienced annually by teachers. The vulnerability of teachers to voice problems has already been discussed but the figures presented only account for those teachers who sought help; many teachers never get as far as the speech and language therapy clinic. For many teachers to admit that they have a problem, which has the potential to affect their ability to teach, would make them feel too vulnerable. Demographic changes in the UK have shown a continuing reduction in the school-age population over successive years, resulting in a concomitant adverse effect on teacher numbers with proportionately fewer teachers being needed, fewer posts being available and therefore greater pressure on those in work to retain their jobs. In this climate teachers who are vocally vulnerable are not likely to advertise the fact by admitting to voice problems, even if there is likely to be a sympathetic response from their head teacher.

When questioned, teachers who have had voice problems reported that when this was brought to the attention of the school there had been support from the relevant authorities (Martin, 1994). There is, however, much anecdotal evidence to suggest that many teachers arrange therapy sessions out of school hours and some never mention the fact that they are undergoing therapy to colleagues or pupils. For those teachers who do not seek help, their only recourse is to try to continue to teach through periods of laryngitis or voice loss – until the next time. For teachers in the USA, the huge cost of health care is often a factor in a teacher's ability to have therapy. If their health insurance does not cover the cost of speech and language therapy, teachers are unable to get help. American teachers have reported that the high cost of insurance was too much for them to sustain and as a result they were effectively unable to do anything other than resign from the profession.

In the UK, information is available from organizations such as The British Voice Association and the Voice Care Network which offers preventive training courses and workshops. Interdisciplinary voice clinics offer treatment from a laryngologist, a speech and language therapist and sometimes an osteopath, an Alexander Technique teacher and a singer. In Sweden, an initiative by the University of Gothenburg offered a voice course where university teachers were given weekly voice training in small groups (Ohlsson, 1993), but this, similar to the University of Warwick's Open Studies programme for professional voice users (Comins, 1995), is the exception rather than the rule.

Many teachers do effect temporary improvement through voice rest, although a significant number of teachers experiencing vocal change simply 'put up with it'. It is unfortunate that, within the population at large, incidents of voice loss or vocal abuse remain a very low priority on the scale of significant illness – indeed there still exists what might be described as a rather *laissez-faire* attitude to voice problems. Vocal dysfunction appears to be something to treat as an occasional 'hazard', rather than attributing it appropriately to the effects of vocal abuse and misuse. Regrettably, this attitude can lead to a spiral of periodic voice loss, followed by periods of remission caused by vocal rest and a gradual acceptance that perhaps the voice is not as good as it was, but it will probably never be any better. Slowly, there is a loss of ability to appraise the voice critically and to notice changes. If proper voice training were given as part of teacher training most teachers would be given the skills to monitor and sustain their own voice effectively throughout their working life. It would also be a much more cost-effective solution to a problem that currently costs education authorities huge sums in lost time and teacher replacements.

This is not to suggest that teachers would never experience voice problems if they were to have training; for a small number of vocally vulnerable teachers problems might still occur, but the numbers would be much reduced. As Sapir et al. (1992) suggest, clinicians have long suspected that lifelong speech habits, such as the tendency to speak rapidly, excessively and/or loudly, may contribute to vocal attrition or the 'wear and tear' of the vocal mechanism, demonstrated by an overall reduction in vocal capabilities associated with acute or chronic abuse or misuse of the phonatory system.

2 The effects of teaching on the voice

Working within the field of occupational voice disorders and specifically in a training role with teachers and lecturers over many years, the authors were aware of the experience of a great many teachers who had previously looked unsuccessfully for, to use their description, 'some sort of support group' for their vocal problems; these individuals had been under the (albeit mistaken) impression that they were the only ones suffering from vocal difficulties. They remarked that, although teacher colleagues seemed to suffer voice loss, this was usually attributed to colds or a virus, with no connection between voice use and voice loss being made. A number of teachers returned for subsequent training because they needed and wanted to retain contact with a group, in order to reassure themselves both that they did have a legitimate problem and that there was a solution.

Much of our early understanding of the complexities of the problems that teachers experience came from those individuals who attended in-service training days; we owe a great deal to them. Women far outnumbered men and this reflected a well-observed gender difference: men generally experience fewer episodes of voice loss than women, resulting partly from their ability to achieve volume without strain, and the greater resonance and therefore carrying power of the male voice. Allied to this is a sociological element; despite attempts to eliminate gender bias, the deeper male voice is often perceived as possessing greater authority and gravitas than the 'lighter' female voice, which, in turn, may contribute to fewer episodes of abusive vocal behaviour. There are, of course, exceptions to every rule and those men who did attend the workshops often appeared more than usually anxious about their voices and under intense stress. Rather than perceiving their vocal problem as a symptom of an occupational disorder, many had internalized the problem, seeing it as caused by some shortcoming within themselves.

What type of training?

The type of voice training required by a teacher is not dissimilar from that required by an actor. The voice is a physical instrument and so training must be given to address not only vocal quality, but also posture and alignment, efficient use of effort, breathing, voice production, projection, 'safe' shouting, interpretative skills and vocal health. The voice, when used efficiently and therefore effectively, can 'work' for as long as necessary without presenting problems, so long as the environmental conditions are reasonable and the voice remains healthy.

A consistent response from teachers (Martin and Darnley, 1996) when questioned about the effects of teaching on the voice was that of vocal tiredness, regardless of whether or not they were encountering vocal problems. Vocal 'tiredness' is neither specific nor easily defined and so to document it here may be naïve, but it was important to explore the opinions of teachers in response to the question 'What are the effects of teaching on your voice?' while accepting that these opinions were, admittedly, subjective. In addition to tiredness, teachers cited 'hoarseness', 'dryness', 'a lack of power', 'an inability to communicate effectively', 'a lack of flexibility', 'a tight and constricted feeling', 'soreness', 'a rasping quality', 'monotony', 'my voice fading after a few hours' and 'feeling that you are stuck on one note'.

Martin (2003) reported that respondents identified a similar list of changes in vocal quality since starting to teach: changes in pitch, huskiness, flexibility, breathiness and harshness, with 56 per cent of respondents noting that their voice had become a little strained, 19 per cent that their voice had become more harsh, 39 per cent that their voice had become slightly husky and 17 per cent that their pitch had lowered. In this study, 23 per cent of respondents noted that their voice had become more flexible since starting to teach, in contrast to the earlier study, where most of the teachers questioned felt that their voices could not operate efficiently over a sustained period of time; a full working day was felt to be too long. At that time, no one reported that their voice had strengthened with use in post, which contrasts with the experience of actors who, with the benefit of voice training, often remark that their voice strengthens over the run of a play, generally building in resonance, flexibility and range.

Many of these descriptions of changes in vocal quality and vocal endurance herald a need for help and indicate changes within either the vocal folds or the structure and functioning of the larynx.

Early warning signals

All voice users should be aware of the following early warning signals and are strongly advised not to dismiss them as 'part of the job', but to seek advice if one or a number occur and do not resolve within a period of 2–3 weeks:

- Recurring loss of voice
- Diminution in range and flexibility
- Pain or discomfort in the area of the larynx
- A marked change in the pitch of the voice after an incident of vocal misuse
- A voice that does not return to normal after a cold or a bout of laryngitis
- Loss of volume with accompanying increase in effort to achieve previous loudness
- A feeling of having a 'lump in the throat'
- Any loss of hearing.

Medical referral

Identifying specific muscles or ligaments is difficult for all but the most skilled, so a voice problem, arising from muscular tension, may often, for example, be interpreted as a 'sore' throat. Teachers reported anecdotally that they had been to their GPs to seek help, but, because they were unable to articulate their voice problem clearly or describe the symptoms with precision, they had left the surgery without the advice and help that they sought.

Within the UK, there are considerable demands on doctors and consequent limits on consultation time, so it is entirely possible that voice problems are not always given the attention that they deserve. On occasions, teachers complained that the doctor's initial response had often been to write out a prescription. This action, however, often distorts the true significance of the problem for the teacher, whose immediate reaction may be to think, 'I'm making a fuss about nothing' or 'It's no wonder my voice is sore, I'm obviously not a good teacher' or 'This is what happens to teachers' voices'.

Teachers report that they consequently feel disinclined to return to the doctor believing that they just have to 'live with it'. Many of the teachers believed that it was not a 'bad enough problem to moan about' in the staff-room or to take time off for. One teacher said:

> It's not like an ankle; when you sprain your ankle everyone can see you are in trouble and they sympathize. No one can see the voice so they often ignore it.

Another teacher said:

> *When my voice is bad, people occasionally say, 'you've got a nasty cold'. I don't bother to explain I don't have a cold at all.*

Another comment frequently heard was:

> *Well you can't really take time off for a bad voice, not like you could for tonsillitis, you don't feel ill when your voice is bad.*

It is to be regretted that, in the experience of those questioned, few doctors appeared willing to refer teachers to a laryngologist or considered reasons other than viral infections for a voice problem.

When attempting to describe the voice problem clearly to the GP it may be useful to think carefully about the aspects outlined below, in order to describe the symptoms more precisely, identify possible triggers and trace the progression of the vocal problem. This in turn will, it is hoped, encourage a more robust response from the GP.

- How long has the problem existed?
- Is it related to a cold or flu?
- Is it linked in any way to an allergic reaction or asthma?
- Can you remember anything that might have precipitated the voice problem, such as shouting or arguing or talking over loud background noise?
- Does it follow a pattern? For example, do you notice it occurring at the same time each day/week/term?
- Is the atmosphere in the classroom dry?
- Have you changed – specifically reduced – the amount of liquid that you drink each day?
- Are you making postural changes in order to accommodate the positioning of the desks, or the height of the blackboard?
- Could your individual teaching style be a contributing factor?
- Do you suffer from backache, neck ache or other physical problems?
- Do you ever get a feeling that you have 'a lump in the throat'?
- Do you feel under professional or personal stress?
- Is there anything you do that helps to reduce the symptoms?

Completion of this personal 'inventory' should allow a clearer picture to emerge of both the onset and the progression of the changes in vocal quality. In this way certain factors, such as aspects of physical health, mental health or environmental factors, may be seen as being implicated in the voice problem.

Describing the symptom

Tiredness

The terminology for voice problems is very subjective, but there are a number of frequently used terms, notably, 'I get hoarse' or 'My voice feels tired', and it would seem to be useful here to describe these terms in more detail. When enquiring further into the 'feelings' of tiredness, comments such as 'My voice gets dry and sore', 'I keep having to swallow', 'It's like there is a tight band around my throat', 'It fades away in the middle of the sentence', 'I have no power', 'I can start off on a reasonable pitch but as I go on it gets higher and higher' may be heard.

This reported 'tiredness' is usually caused by ineffective production of the voice. The muscles used to produce sound are used in other functions, such as lifting, pushing, giving birth, coughing and keeping foreign bodies from getting into the lungs. As they possess an innate muscularity, they are also capable of being inadvertently over-used in the production of voice. Muscle tension disorders (where there is increased tension in the neck and suprahyoid muscles), with muscle aches and fatigue, are a well-known effect of vocal misuse and abuse. When used efficiently, the voice does not tire. When used without proper breath support and with poorly aligned body posture, and when more muscles than those necessary for the purpose are used, the voice begins to tire.

Hoarseness/huskiness

In the perceptual description of voice quality the terms 'husky' and 'hoarse' are often combined, because they do not stand particularly successfully on their own. Associated with breathiness, tension and strain there is generally a rather low, rough, as distinct from breathy, sound. Hoarseness occurs because the vocal folds are only partly vibrated along their full length, as a result of being swollen. It is not necessarily accompanied by any pain or discomfort, although it may be. The voice in this condition is sometimes described as attractive or even 'sexy' and, because of this, sufferers may fail to rest the voice to reduce swelling and allow the vocal folds to return to their natural state.

Dehydration may be another possible reason for the hoarse/husky vocal quality. The vocal folds need to be well hydrated in order to withstand the intense demands of prolonged voice use. It is important to build up hydration levels in the body and thus hydrate the tissue and membrane of the vocal tract. Classrooms are frequently artificially dry and overheated. Teachers are often discouraged from drinking during class, not only because of perceived health and safety risks imposed by the school, but also quite prosaically because the result of drinking more means leaving the classroom and going to the lavatory. Recent concern about the levels of dehydration among pupils, leading to reduced concentration and learning ability, has, however, increased attention on levels of hydration, and it is hoped that improved focus on this will have a correspondingly beneficial effect for teachers. As a rough 'rule of thumb', the more an individual has to speak, the more he or she should drink, but it is important to remember that this does not achieve an instant response – introduce increased levels of hydration in the form of water gradually. Tea, coffee and some forms of carbonated drinks have dehydrating properties and alcohol is particularly drying. Many people when asked whether they drink enough will respond that they do, only to discover that, although they are drinking, they are drinking liquids of the 'wrong' kind.

Similar vocal symptoms may be experienced with laryngitis: in extreme cases the voice may vanish altogether or diminish to a whisper. Teachers, as already noted, tend to 'soldier on', ignoring the problem. Ignoring the problem is not to be encouraged because, when the vocal folds are swollen and closure is incomplete, the muscles of the larynx have to overwork to produce a sound. The volume required to reach the back of the classroom or, worse still, to control a group of noisy children on the sports field results in real strain and can, in severe cases, damage the folds.

It is possible that an allergic reaction may be responsible for the hoarse quality. This can be related to hay fever or pollution allergies, and can result in either a reduction in the lubrication of the vocal folds or an abundance of mucus. Asthma, with its consequential effect of reducing lung capacity, can contribute to vocal strain and hoarseness. It is often misplaced stoicism that encourages a teacher to continue under these conditions: the voice in this state is seldom effective. The husky voice can have the effect of making an audience feel tired and inattentive. The emotional edge to the voice has gone and the tension that goes into producing the sound becomes the quality that is listened to. It is interesting to observe an audience being addressed by a 'hoarse' speaker; they often clear their throats in sympathy or even cough.

What causes hoarseness?

If there is no cold or infection, there is probably a functional reason for the hoarse sound of the voice. It could be that the individual's posture is not conducive to easy, efficient production of the voice, so that the muscles overwork, resulting in 'strain'. In an otherwise healthy voice, there is usually a fairly easily correctable reason for the problem, which is very often linked to breathing. A fuller description of breathing is given in Chapter 4, but it is important to say here that the breath is responsible for the vibration of the folds and, if that breath is either not powerful enough to set the folds in motion or not synchronized with the activity of voice, problems can occur. Breath is closely linked to the emotional life of us all and so when we are under stress we are more likely to 'block' or inhibit the very natural and normal activity of breathing.

The teacher's perspective

A small-scale, in-depth study conducted by means of a questionnaire (Martin and Darnley, 1996) allowed for an exploration of some of the problems that teachers encountered in terms of how their own voices 'performed' under teaching conditions, and how confident or otherwise they were with their own level of language use. The study was conducted in a primary school, in a residential area, with no major discipline problems among the children aged from rising 5 to 11 years. A hearing unit attached to the school meant that hearing-impaired children were integrated into the school. There were children with other special needs within the school, but these represented a small percentage of the school population.

Of the staff who completed the questionnaire, 78 per cent had no work on their voice during their training, 87 per cent said that their voice had failed at some point in their professional life, becoming croaky, hoarse or husky, and 21 per cent of those questioned said that their voice had disappeared altogether. When asked 'Does your throat ever get tight?', 87 per cent said yes and 65 per cent said that they thought that this was a common complaint. Despite the difficulties that they experienced with their voices, 88 per cent said that it conveyed the qualities that they wanted to convey, but when asked to describe their voice some of the adjectives used were, 'squeaky', 'quite weak', 'loud', 'husky', 'creaky', 'low pitched'. Only 22 per cent were happy with their voice as it was. When asked to name the most difficult vocal situation that they encountered, 'parents' evenings' were named by 34 per cent of the teachers, with 23 per cent citing 'reprimanding the class' as the most difficult vocal situation.

The teachers were asked if they saw themselves as performers and all those questioned said 'yes'. When asked how confident they were with spoken language, 65 per cent said that they were confident, but, when asked if their confidence would be the same with a different age group, only 22 per cent said 'yes'. When asked what aspects of teaching they were not fully prepared for in college, their answers ranged from drama and story-telling, the pastoral role of a teacher, the stamina required, the work levels, to the amount of talking, the use of the voice and behaviour management skills.

This study looked at results from one primary school, but a subsequent study (Martin, 2003) gathered responses from a postal questionnaire sent to newly qualified primary teachers and lecturers in further education, in over 60 different locations. Although very different in both structure and range, many of the results obtained mirrored the earlier findings in that issues of voice loss, changes in vocal quality, lack of vocal robustness, anxiety and concern about vocal health all featured highly.

As has already been noted, studies worldwide have shown similar patterns of vocal attrition. Could it be said that voice problems within the teaching profession have reached epidemic proportions?

There is no typical teacher, but the following case histories are included to offer a more personal insight into the human face of these statistics.

Case study: Avril

An example of the impact that the demands of teaching make on the voice is seen in the case of Avril. Avril is 38 years old, a mother of three who is married to a man whose job involves her in a considerable amount of entertaining and socializing. Avril is therefore accustomed to using her voice in a social setting and often among large noisy groups. Deciding to retrain as a teacher Avril enrolled on a Postgraduate Certificate in Education (PGCE) course. Before her marriage she had trained as a specialist teacher of speech and drama and had also worked as a professional actress in a touring educational theatre group. This work had been both tiring and demanding vocally, but she had her training and technique to draw on. The company often performed twice and sometimes three times a day and travelled great distances between schools. As the plays were participatory, she was involved in controlling the often very large groups but never experienced any vocal problems. After her period with the Theatre in Education group she performed in musicals and rock operas, again never experiencing vocal difficulties. A period of 15 years elapsed, during which she left the theatre and worked as a personal assistant in broadcasting and had her three children. She stopped working on her voice during this time, but kept herself physically fit by working out in a gymnasium and doing aerobic exercises.

Once she found herself in the classroom she was amazed and rather shocked to find that at the end of the day her voice felt tired and sore. 'I felt as if I would develop nodules if I didn't do something about it,' she said. 'I realized I must go back to working on my breathing because I never had these problems when I acted.' Asked why she thought this was so, she replied: 'When you are acting you are very aware of technique. Breath support is part of the job and is integrated into the performance.

My teaching practice took place in a school where discipline was a problem. I found myself constantly having to reprimand the children. My actions were spontaneous and I suppose I felt out of control at times. I had lost my objectivity and my reactions were subjective.'

With someone who has previously experienced the ability to support the voice, it is easy to remind him or her of the sensations and to help him or her to re-establish healthy usage. As Avril had kept fit and in touch with her body, her breathing muscles did not take long to re-establish their previous tone. Avril recognized the effect on her voice of stress, which in her case was related to the additional work and organization involved in doing first her BA degree and then the PGCE. As so often happens with a mature student, she had taken her studies extremely seriously and achieved excellent grades. In addition, however, she had had to juggle her children's needs, both practical and emotional, with the social demands of her husband's career, running the home and finding time to study.

Case study: Theresa

Another interesting case is that of Theresa. We met her when she became aware of her need to address her vocal problem. She had a history of recurring voice loss and sounded husky even when her voice was at its best. She is not a smoker but described her voice as sounding like that of a heavy smoker. She noticed that her voice was at its worst after a night in the pub, after singing or talking for sustained periods.

The most impressive and appealing quality about Theresa is her natural exuberance; she is enormously positive and personable and constantly 'on the go' – her energy seems boundless. As a single mother she has to cope with stress, and her coping strategy is to meet life's challenges 'head on', but her personal strength is also the reason her tensions are manifested in her voice. Her energy emanates from the neck and shoulder area and, although she is able to relax given time, she does not do so easily. Her breath is shallow and she tends to hold onto it, rather than to release it into voice and speech. Her habitual head/neck alignment is to position her head in front of her shoulders, leading to considerable strain on the muscles of the neck and shoulders, and therefore the laryngeal structure is under stress. She speaks loudly and rapidly, and complains of dryness and a feeling of tightness in the larynx. Her general effort level is high.

Theresa is an excellent example of the important relationship between physicality and the voice. There is nothing wrong with her voice but the stresses and strains that non-alignment of the spine, shoulders, neck and head have placed on her larynx, plus the overwork that she forces on her laryngeal muscles, have produced a set of circumstances that she perceives as a 'voice' problem. Add to this the poor use of breath and the emotional stresses involved with being a single working mother, and the result is that her voice is 'under attack'.

To counter these problems, Theresa has enormous resources. She has the intelligence to perceive that all is not well and has the will and ability to do something about it. She is a pliable individual open to change. She has had counselling from a qualified therapist over the break-up of her relationship with her child's father, and has a great deal of self-knowledge and motivation. The enthusiasm that produced the problem is the best weapon that she has to deal with it.

Case study: Hazel

Hazel is an art student whom we met while she was working as a dresser at one of the London theatres. Hazel had been a teacher for 10 years but had been forced to give up work because she developed vocal nodules. The progression from a healthy voice at the beginning of her career to a voice unable to cope with the demands of the profession was a fairly lengthy process. Vocal nodules begin as soft, small, red swellings on the edges of the vocal folds, but in time without treatment they will harden, become fibrous and white in colour. With early treatment and attention to good vocal hygiene and usage, they will disappear, but if left untreated they often require surgical removal, as in Hazel's case.

Two issues, which she highlighted as contributing factors, were that she was working as a primary school teacher with 7-year-old Bangladeshi children in an open plan school. The children were naturally very vocal and as a teacher she admits that she encouraged quite a noisy working environment, partly because there was a need for the children to speak in order to progress in English, so the more talking that went on the better, and also, as the children were naturally noisy, she liked to encourage them to be noisy and she enjoyed a noisy, busy environment. The open plan class arrangement meant that there were noises from the other classes, so in order to be heard Hazel had to raise her voice over the ambient noise in addition to the noise of the 30 children whom she was teaching. The general noise level was high because there were no partitions between classes, just pillars to define the space.

In addition to her teaching load Hazel used to work with puppets, for which she had not had any formal training. The effect on her voice from postural factors was considerable as she moved from standing to crouching positions, and of course she often spoke with her head tipped back. As well as this less than ideal position for voicing, she also told us that she spoke regularly to children at a distance, raising her voice to do so.

As Hazel said: 'You are encouraged to talk all the time from 9am to 3:30pm, using a raised pitch for nearly all this time.' Hazel took water into the classroom, but generally water in the classroom was not encouraged and there was no water near the radiator or any attempt to humidify the room. Hazel reported there had been no help or advice about looking after her voice or any suggestion that she should be aware of it when she was training. At college she was simply told 'Your voice is your control' so there were no strategies on offer to help students; indeed, she said that it was 'all a question of luck'.

In Hazel's case there was no evidence of vocal vulnerability as either a student or a teacher. She had enjoyed working in the noisy, lively environment of the school, which she admitted was quite stressful but very friendly, and it had taken her a long time to realize that there was a real problem with her voice, which initially became husky. She subsequently realized that she needed to use a lot of effort to talk and could not get volume. For a while she lost her voice completely. Realizing that there was a problem, she went to her doctor who fortunately took it seriously and referred her to a specialist straight away. Hazel was lucky in that the school was most supportive and she was able to have an appointment time at 4pm, which meant that she only missed the last half-hour of school. Hazel said that the problem that many teachers experience is the feeling of guilt when taking time off. There was no budget at her school to cover supply teaching, so if she took a day off funds for a supply teacher were used which could otherwise have gone to replace equipment or buy some item that was much needed. Teachers at her school made every effort to go into school unless desperately ill. Equally, she reported that there was already so much time taken out of the school week by paper work, testing of children and meetings, that there was a great desire on the part of all staff to minimize the time spent away.

Hazel was fortunate in that she was able to go on to art college and retrain, because otherwise her voice problems would have meant that she would have had to take 6 months off. Hazel agreed that she had always taken her voice for granted, never bothered about it and in her words 'produced it haphazardly'. The year that her voice became a problem was the first year of the National Curriculum, which increased her workload dramatically. Another contributory factor, she felt, was that 95 per cent of the school population was Asian in an area that was adjacent to a district with elected members of the British National Front on the district council. This created considerable stress within the area, although Hazel said that there were no discipline problems at her school. Hazel agreed that this extreme external social stress was possibly a contributory factor, because environmental factors are closely linked to vocal abuse and misuse.

In looking at factors such as diet, Hazel said that she used to eat very spicy food but did not eat late at night and did not drink, although she regularly smoked 10 cigarettes a day and had done so from the age of 15. She stopped smoking when her voice problems were identified.

On a personal level Hazel found that her loss of voice was very distressing; not only was it quite painful to talk but it was amazingly debilitating. As a teacher she had become used to 'arranging' things with her voice, which she likened to conducting. She had 'conducted' with her voice, and felt completely helpless and feeble without it. Her voice had been like a tool, one that she suddenly could not use. At the end of each day she was really tired and felt quite ill: she found it difficult to breathe and the strain of speaking all the time was very taxing. It seemed to her as though she was talking at the top of her voice, yet only a small sound was emerging and quite often she could not speak at all. Hazel had voice therapy for almost a year. During this time she could not talk at night and as a result she stopped going out. She said that she felt very isolated because there is great pressure to speak in company and, when she could not do so comfortably, she got quite depressed.

Her experience of voice loss was one of isolation and distress, with accompanying periods of depression. Eventually Hazel's voice returned but she had to leave the profession because her voice would not have supported the demands of a teaching career. Even now Hazel still has periods of vocal strain if she talks in clubs and pubs over noise, so she remains vigilant about avoiding situations that may be vocally taxing. She will 'warm-up' now if she is going to have to talk for any length of time, and drinks a lot of water, drinking herbal teas in preference to coffee or tea, and she uses steam if she has been misusing her voice. Hazel commented that, when she lost her voice, she felt as though she was 'shut into a box' and could not communicate. She was aware of being treated differently in shops, and social occasions were an enormous pressure. The invisibility of her injury was difficult, as was the uncertainty of achieving voice, because there was no certainty before she spoke that she would be able to produce sound. In addition she reported that, when she lost her voice initially, she did not know if it would ever come back, which made her incredibly anxious.

Hazel's experience is one that must be familiar to many readers and is perhaps a useful illustration of the effects of teaching on one teacher's voice. This exciting and imaginative teacher is now lost to the profession. More specific help during her 3-year training course could have avoided the problems that she encountered.

3 The effect on the voice of external stress factors

Stress at work

Powell (1997) suggests that work stress is the single most important cause of stress. He evidences a study of financial institutions in which 64 per cent of employers regarded excessive stress as the principal health threat facing the company. In 1999 the Department of Health reported stress at work reaching epidemic proportions (Milne, 1999). It was recognized as the biggest occupational health problem with up to 6 million working days lost a year at a cost of about £5 billion (Milne, 1999). In a Trades Union Congress survey of 8000 health and safety union representatives, three-quarters described stress as a major hazard compared with two-thirds in 1997 (Milne, 1999).

Stress defined

In any discussion of stress it is important to try to define what is understood by the term 'stress' and that in itself presents a problem, as noted by Travers and Cooper (1996). Tension, strain and pressure are words that may be used synonymously with 'stress' whereas stress may be seen paradoxically as both negative and positive. Stress affects everyone but not to the same extent. Stress is a necessary and essential part of human life, and may therefore be described as a form of interaction between the environmental demands and the individual's ability to meet those demands.

Each individual has a unique response to stress; stress perceived by one as beneficial and stimulating, inspiring the individual to perform well, may be perceived as too much by another, and thus his or her ability to perform well will be impaired. For the individual who responds to stress positively, too little stress can in fact reduce effectiveness and leave the individual listless and under-stimulated.

Prevalence of teacher stress

Given that work stress has reached a critical level within the work place, and in recognition of the effect of stress on the voice, it is important to examine the prevalence of stress among the teaching profession. In addition, it is vital to acknowledge the extent to which a teacher's working environment contributes to teacher stress.

The prevalence of teacher stress is a worldwide phenomenon, which had already been identified almost three decades ago. Coates and Thoresen (1976) suggested that the number of teachers experiencing high levels of perceived stress was as high as 70 per cent, whereas Dunham (1983) reported a figure of 30 per cent.

In 1992, *The Independent* reported that:

> *The number of retirements due to ill health increased from 1,617 in 1979/80 to 4,123 in 1989/90, with a large jump in 1988 when the Education Reform Act brought in the National Curriculum.*
>
> 25th January 1991, as quoted in Travers and Cooper (1996)

Such was the concern about the level of stress experienced by teachers within the UK that the second largest teaching union, the National Association of Schoolmasters/Union of Women Teachers (NASUWT), commissioned a comprehensive study of teacher stress (Travers and Cooper, 1993); the findings indicated that teachers, compared with other highly stressed occupational groups, experienced lower job satisfaction and poorer mental health. Teachers were found to be reporting stress-related manifestations that were far higher than the population norms and of other comparable occupational groups. Travers and Cooper (1993) discovered that the major areas of job dissatisfaction were the job pressure factors of 'management/structure of the school' and 'lack of status and promotion'.

In 1999 the British Government sponsored a helpline for teachers, Teacherline (Lightfoot, 1999), which was expected to offer advice to a predicted 15,000 teachers each year. Launching the helpline, the then Minister of State for Education said:

> *... it is not a Government initiative because we put so much pressure on teachers but one which comes from the profession itself ...*

The need for this initiative, irrespective of by whom or why it was set up, would seem to indicate that little has changed over the past three decades with regard to levels of teacher stress. This would seem to be confirmed by the award to a teacher of a quarter of a million pounds for a stress-related compensation claim (Owen, 2002). At about the same time, the then general secretary of the NASUWT was reported to have said that the union was dealing with 120 stress-related compensation claims; he predicted that unless action was taken there could be thousands more teachers with a valid claim (Owen, 2002).

Changes within the education sector in the UK, be it in primary, secondary or tertiary education, have been frequent and numerous and have contributed substantially to the stress experienced by teachers in the work place (Coopers and Lybrand Deloitte, 1994; Evans et al., 1994; Cains, 1995). Wu's study (1998) confirmed this, reporting on 'changes in education in recent years which have brought about tremendous pressure on teachers'.

It is not within the scope of this book to itemize the changes or comment on the political, demographic, financial and social factors for these changes. It is, however, important to look at educational change in the context of the individual teacher working within this environment, and who is subject to the inherent tensions and stress that accompany change.

Occupational stress

The prevailing feeling within the teaching profession in the UK is one of low morale and poor self-image. Blunkett (1998), in his role as Minister of State for Education, claimed that 'there is . . . too much poor or inadequate teaching'. It is therefore perhaps no surprise to note that a survey published by the National Union of Teachers (NUT) in January 2000 reported that most primary teachers say that they feel demoralized, overworked and undervalued (Carvel, 2000).

In addition, teachers are known to be overwhelmed with work. Teachers see initiative overload from successive governments and agencies as being at the root of the problem, allied to the huge increases in bureaucracy and the mountain of paper work that this generates. Also teachers and lecturers have found that they are expected to take on greater and greater responsibility after very little time in teaching (Martin, 2003). Posts of special responsibility, after-school activities, league sports teams, music or drama events, and the integration of special needs children within mainstream schooling, all create additional pressures for the teacher. As a result teachers are, in increasing numbers, bowing out. Figures published by the National Association of Head Teachers reported in 1994 that, since the early 1980s, the number of teachers ending their careers early because of ill-health trebled in the UK, with only one teacher in five working on to the statutory retirement age.

In 1998, the Teacher Training Agency, in an effort to raise recruitment, introduced a £5000 'golden hello' for mathematics and science trainees, followed in 2000 by a UK Government scheme which paid £6000 salaries to trainee teachers in a similar drive to encourage graduates to become teachers (Charter, 2000). Despite this, however, in 2002, Ofsted's annual report found there were still real problems, not only in recruiting but also in retaining teachers, with 20 per cent of teachers leaving within their first 3 years in the profession; heavy workload was cited as one of the reasons for leaving. Overall, 74 per cent of teachers leaving primary schools and 58 per cent leaving secondary schools gave workload as a reason (Smithers and Robinson, 2003).

It is, however, encouraging to note that major Government changes to teachers' pay and conditions in England and Wales, *Raising standards and tackling work-load: a national agreement* (DfES, 2003), as agreed with all but one of the teacher and support staff unions, should mean that all teachers in England and Wales have a reasonable balance between work and non-work life by 2005. The effect of this should be to reduce teachers' working week below the current average of 52 hours and to increase the proportion of the working week spent teaching and preparing.

Physiological effects of stress

Stress may be seen to be an adaptive response by the body to changes in the environment, e.g. if confronted by a man-eating lion, most individuals would be activated by an instinctive response either to turn and run away, or to stand and fight. Although evolutionary changes have made it less likely that individuals will meet many lions, the response to potentially threatening situations remains the same and the primitive body in a state of high alert prepares to use reserves of energy to 'fight or flee'.

The threat of physical, emotional and psychological pain is ever present, if not actually encountered, and on occasions the 'fight-or-flight' response is triggered without the individual being fully aware of it, but physiological change will have taken place nevertheless. It is that physiological change that has, both directly and indirectly, an effect on the vocal process.

Some of the physiological changes that occur as the body, responding to the threat, 'prepares for action', regardless of how dramatic or otherwise this action is, are listed here:

- The pupils dilate and the mouth goes dry
- Neck and shoulder muscles tense
- The large skeletal muscles contract for action
- Breathing becomes faster and shallower
- The heart pumps blood faster so that blood vessels dilate
- The liver releases stored sugar to provide fuel for quick energy
- Digestion slows down or ceases

- Muscles at the opening of the bladder and anus are relaxed
- Cortisol, adrenaline and noradrenaline are released.

When the source of the threat is removed or resolved, the body returns to a stable state or homeostasis. However, in a period of prolonged stress individuals may activate the stress response but cannot activate the accompanying physical response, becoming impatient, angry and irritated instead. They therefore do not return to a homeostatic state and it is in the inhibition of the physical response to stress that the danger to health lies. The individual may well continue to demonstrate many of the symptoms below in the absence of any threat:

- difficulty in swallowing
- aching neck
- backache
- muscle tension
- muscle pain
- fatigue
- frequent urination and diarrhoea
- less efficient immune system
- over-breathing
- indigestion.

The effect of stress on the voice

The interrelationship of voice, emotion and physical state has been clearly established for many years, as seen in the seminal work by Moses (1954), *The Voice of Neurosis*, although this information is possibly less well known by the public at large. Voice is a very critical indicator of both physiological and psychological well-being and as such offers a particularly acute and effective gauge of physical and mental health. In effect the voice is a very precise stress indicator. A rather obvious but pertinent example is the way in which an individual's mood may be judged on the telephone. There are no indicators other than the voice to help identify mood – no facial expression, body posture or gesture – yet mood, emotion and physical state will be illustrated by the initial greeting. Energy levels, mood and physical health are reflected in the voice.

Many of the stress-induced physical changes that have been described above will have a significant effect on voice quality. Reviewing these physical changes reveals a clear link between voice and stress:

- Difficulty in swallowing leads to a fixed laryngeal position.

- Aching neck leads to tension within the internal and external muscles of the larynx.
- Backache affects the easy movement of the ribs.
- Muscle tension affects the easy movement of the ribs.
- Muscle tension reduces the flexibility and muscularity of the respiratory process.
- Muscle pain leads to reduced voluntary movement, resulting in stiffness and loss of flexibility.
- Fatigue leads to loss of effective muscle function.
- Frequent urination and diarrhoea lead to dehydration and a consequent effect on the vocal folds.
- A less efficient immune system leads to lowered resistance to upper respiratory tract infections and potential for infection within the larynx.
- Over-breathing leads to a reduction in both breath support and phonation time.
- Indigestion may lead to gastro-oesophageal reflux, which will directly affect the vocal folds, causing redness and irritation.

Examination of these physical changes in the light of the processes that affect voice illustrates the fact that stress may affect every aspect of phonation, including breath capacity, muscle function, reduced lubrication of the vocal folds, changes within the lining of the vocal tract and tissue integrity of the vocal folds. Although noting the physiological changes caused by stress, it is also important to recognize that the physical changes that occur in a state of low esteem will also contribute to vocal change. Here the most noticeable changes are often postural, with lowered eye levels, slumped shoulders, rounded back and a much more contained, introverted posture, with accumulated tension in the shoulders, neck and jaw.

These cumulative changes, both physiological and psychological, occurring as a result of stress, will often have the effect of making the individual feel exhausted and unable to function effectively. Later chapters explore language use within the teaching environment, but it is important to note that, although the focus here has been on the effect of stress on vocal quality, the use and retrieval of language may also be affected. Continually being studied and defined and not yet completely understood, language is a highly complicated process, paradoxically most vividly illustrated when there is a breakdown in the structure when, for example, an individual has a 'stroke'. The expression 'I was so tired that I could hardly say a word', more usually thought of as referring to the physical process of articulation, also encompasses the cognitive processes involved in 'saying a word'. The forgetting of perfectly simple words or losing the train of thought is often aggravated by tiredness and, in some instances, tension and stress.

Coping with change

Education is a dynamic political arena, the focus of Government initiatives and funding, but for those at all levels within education this dynamism can also be the focus of tension and stress. Teachers experience a sense of dislocation because the framework within which they teach changes. Syllabus changes will mean that teachers have suddenly to learn new material and often feel uncomfortable with the short period of time that they are given to assimilate it. Teachers who are qualified to teach one subject find themselves having to teach another with which they are comparatively unfamiliar, having to keep one step ahead of the class. This is not to suggest that teachers want to collude in apparently offering less than expert tuition, but simply that limits imposed by the pupil:staff ratio and the subject choices made by pupils mean that this does occur. The level of tension that is engendered is considerable; most teachers want to be prepared, to be confident about the subject and to feel that they can legitimately be 'the expert'. The difficulty for teachers lies in trying to reconcile the demands of the school administration and their own needs, and on most occasions the requirements of the school take precedence.

Within a small-scale study of newly qualified teachers and lecturers (Martin, 2003), respondents reported that they had been asked to take on additional posts of special responsibility, for which they felt unprepared. If one assumes that this is not an isolated case, there must be many teachers struggling to maintain their position against overwhelming administrative and professional demands. In addition to these professional demands, teachers are not immune to the effects of stress within their personal lives, e.g. bereavement, miscarriage, divorce, redundancy of a partner and prolonged chronic illness, which do not prevent them from teaching but do have a very debilitating effect.

In addition to voice problems relating to illness, teachers frequently report voice problems related to classroom discipline or indeed to incidents with individual pupils. Teachers suddenly experience voice problems that they can directly relate to difficulty with a particular pupil; their perception is that, as they became more stressed by the situation, so they experienced voice problems.

As has already been noted, for some individuals stress is stimulating and exciting, whereas for others a similar degree of stress is unbearable and can result in sleeplessness, depression, anxiety attacks or a vocal problem. Both responses activate (as part of the fight-or-flight response) the release of large amounts of adrenaline and noradrenaline, which help individuals maintain a high level of activity, giving that extra 'buzz' that people experience when working at full stretch. The effect, however, of unusually high levels of noradrenaline ultimately leads to an abrupt loss of energy, often accompanied by an overwhelming feeling of exhaustion unrelated to physical effort. Some teachers experience this effect at the end of every term; for others, this is an occasional episode triggered when the cumulative effects of personal and professional stress become too much.

Changes in vocal quality

The effect of stress on the voice has already been outlined; the tired and strained vocal quality with which teachers present at the end of term is a well-known phenomenon in staff-rooms all over the world. So, too, is the fact that many teachers experience problems at the beginning of the autumn term when returning after a long summer break. One reason for this may be that, during the summer holiday period, teachers have been able to effect some form of 'damage limitation' as far as the voice is concerned. Periods of speaking with less effort and in a more vocally friendly environment allow the voice to return to a more natural vocal setting. The teacher returns to the school environment still using this 'holiday' vocal setting, but may soon find that the voice is inadequate for the task and there is a need to readjust and adapt to the school/college environment.

Our individual response to stress and tension cannot be absolutely anticipated; we can predict danger areas but we do not know definitely what the effects will be. Some teachers can demonstrate amazing vocal resilience for years, only to find that their voice disappears without any apparent increase in vocal loading, whereas other teachers experience mild vocal symptoms for years that never get any worse or become unmanageable. What is known, however, is that most teachers and indeed most voice patients will report the same feelings: diminution of vocal flexibility, range, loudness or ease of voicing leads to an erosion of their concept of self. The inability to express feelings, emotions and thoughts properly because of voice loss caused by vocal abuse or misuse is very alienating.

Environmental factors

How can teachers better anticipate factors that will increase the likelihood of vocal strain? Potential stress triggers and identified emotional and physical factors that can affect voice quality have already been discussed; Chapter 8 explores ways in which the voice can be protected.

The influence of environmental factors as a source of stress may, however, be overlooked. It is important that teachers acknowledge the influence of the environment in which they work on their mental health – issues such as overcrowding and lack of personal space within the school.

Well-documented evidence shows that where individuals have to live and work in overcrowded conditions the levels of tension rise, and this increase is reflected in heightened feelings of aggression and violence. For many teachers, issues of overcrowding are considered only in terms of class size. Increases in class size are cited as giving teachers problems related to actual teaching efficiency. How can you teach 40 children in one class? How can you respond to the needs of every child? How can you keep control? There is also the issue of overcrowding and psychological response. It is clear that, if one adds feelings of tension arising from overcrowding to the difficulty of controlling large numbers of children, the resulting cocktail is fairly potent.

Teachers deserve to have some professional advice in terms of the new developments in ergonomics and to try to limit problems of overcrowding, if at all possible. Apart from the central issue of too many people in too small a space, it is also important to look at the effect that it has on the pupils who are equally influenced by the space in which they work. Teachers report on the negative effect that the absence of a designated personal space has – particularly a problem for those in further education who are contracted not to a college, but to an agency, or those individuals who work as supply teachers.

Although children have an opportunity to release tension in a physical way through play and sports sessions, teachers have limited opportunity to do the same. The environment in which an individual works or learns has a powerful influence on mood and emotion, one that should be considered more robustly.

Time management

The importance of achieving a satisfactory work/life balance has received considerable attention in the last decade and it is acknowledged that teachers work more intensively than people in other occupations, with 50- to 60-hour weeks the norm. Head teachers reportedly work 300–400 hours more per annum than similar managers and professionals (PricewaterhouseCoopers, cited in Berliner, 2003).

Time management and task prioritization are key strategies in response to a growing recognition of the increased and unacceptable level of work overload within many different working arenas in the UK. Yet they are very difficult to achieve without help. Working with another person to look at issues of concern is important, but so often the most recurring theme is lack of time. Something as simple as list making, a different method of filing, a memo or day book in which to write all tasks and carry forward those that have not been completed to the next day, will greatly help the administrative aspects of life that can become so overwhelming. Another supremely effective method is to learn to say 'no', taking care that this decision does not simply shift the load from you to another colleague with equal workload and responsibilities.

Workshops on time management are to be recommended as a productive way of spending in-service funds, empowering the teacher to make constructive changes to his or her personal and working environment.

4 How the voice works

Voice, the process that changes silent thought into spoken word, is, for most people, something that just happens – the mouth opens to verbalize thoughts and voice occurs spontaneously. You think of something to say, you say it, and how it actually happens is a matter of some conjecture, if indeed it is thought of at all. That is until something goes wrong and, even then, the mechanics of voice production are generally ignored and the most usually cited 'cure-all' is either a hot drink with honey and lemon to 'soothe' the voice, or a period without talking to 'rest' the voice.

More often, however, the individual concerned struggles on with faint cries of 'It will get better by itself, just give it a few days' and usually that is exactly what happens. The previously husky voice improves spontaneously, the individual heaves a sigh of relief and keeps on using the voice in exactly the same way – until the next time. Indeed, if the individual concerned is a teacher, there may be an opportunity for voice rest in the form of a half-term break or weekend. On Monday the voice seems a lot better, so back the teacher goes, reporting to colleagues that all is now well – until the next time, and inevitably there will be a next time.

Misuse and abuse of the voice

It is difficult to think of any other injury that individuals pay as little attention to as a voice injury. In general, if experiencing muscle strain, back problems, a broken leg or a sprained wrist, the tendency is to say 'must be careful and not do that again', taking care when next in the same situation to avoid the problem. With voice disorders, however, how often is there any attempt to try to avoid the same situation? In a smoky atmosphere or a dusty, noisy environment, rather than immediately making a fast exit in order to preserve voice, the individual concerned will generally 'sit tight', rationalizing his or her actions by saying, 'it would seem anti-social if I left, I will probably be fine after a night's sleep, perhaps I will get used to it after a while'. Rather than sit mutely by and not talk over a high noise level, individuals continue to shout over the band, and struggle home complaining of sore throats and voices that rasp perilously out of control from treble to bass.

So why does this vocal misuse and abuse continue to occur? If an individual with a large bruise on his or her leg were seen banging against it with the other leg or hitting an injured arm with a fist, this behaviour would be seen as somewhat bizarre. So what makes the voice so prone to self-inflicted vandalism? Part of the answer must lie in the fact that the damage sustained by the vocal folds cannot be seen and thus individuals remain supremely indifferent to any suggestion that damage is occurring. The voice that is slightly husky and breathy as a result of injury is described, as already noted, as 'sexy' rather than vulnerable. Indeed, many people prefer a vocal quality that is low in pitch, as an overly high pitch is sometimes perceived as shrill and unpleasant to listen to, so the 'injured' low voice can often pass without comment.

A sign hung at the front door of every teaching institution emblazoned with the words 'You are now entering a voice watch zone' would usefully serve to highlight the vocal problems endemic to school life.

The mechanics of voice

So what does happen within the larynx and why may it be of interest to readers? Certainly the authors are not advocating an intimate knowledge of the larynx as a prerequisite for all professional voice users. A too scrupulous concern for what is happening within the larynx can sometimes inhibit vocal freedom and limit the expressivity of the voice – a very necessary component for a professional voice user. It is, however, essential that the professional voice user be secure in the knowledge that his or her voice is efficient, effective and reliable. To achieve this, it is necessary to be aware of and knowledgeable about one's own voice, to understand its strengths and limitations, to predict vocal demands and to adjust voice use accordingly. Through the delivery of more training and increased vocal health education provision this could be achieved.

In the same way that some individuals can run without tiring for miles, whereas others wilt after the first half-mile, so, with the voice, some individuals are less vocally robust than others – they cannot easily sustain extended periods of speech. There is therefore a need to recognize one's vocal limitations and avoid situations that exacerbate problems. Perhaps a useful analogy is that of driving a car. It may not be possible to name each individual component in the engine, but it is possible to listen to the noise of the engine and recognize when there is a need to change gear. Hazards placed on the route ahead are avoided. In the same way, it is important to learn to listen and monitor vocal quality, identify trouble spots and avoid dangers, to hear when a voice is being strained and in this way recognize and avoid situations that are vocally hazardous.

Each one of us has a voice that is unique, one that can be instantly identified as belonging to us by those whom we know. We can affect vocal change, in terms of altering volume, speed and pitch, while still retaining the unique qualities that identify it as our voice. In this chapter, the structure of the larynx and the vocal process is described in considerable detail in order to provide a resource for those readers who, out of interest or because they are experiencing difficulty, want more detailed information on vocal structure and function.

Knowledge of the function and structure of the vocal process is not a prerequisite of good voice, but for many it does help to promote more effective use of voice and encourage vocal hygiene and conservation.

How voice is produced

Voice production is dependent on three different systems:

1. The respiratory system responsible for the manner and pattern of breathing
2. The phonatory system responsible for how sound is produced within the larynx
3. The resonatory system responsible for modification of this sound

These separate systems have been adapted to work together in the process of voice production, although their primary biological purpose is of course to assist in life support. Without air we would die, without the closure of the vocal folds to sustain subglottic pressure we would find it much more difficult to lift heavy articles or push down, e.g. in defecation or childbirth, and without the epiglottis closing over the trachea food or liquid would enter the lungs and we could choke. When food does 'go down the wrong way', the lungs try to expel it as quickly as possible and we cough violently.

Although the systems are interdependent, voice is the result of a combined effort by all three. What must also be remembered is that these systems are directly affected by posture. Virtually every bone in the body forms a joint or is connected to some other bone, allowing freedom of movement, but it also means that movement of one body part will affect another either directly or indirectly. The interrelationship of head, neck and back, and what happens to the positioning of the spine and pelvis, will affect the ribcage and consequently respiration and voicing. For this reason, when we think of voice work we need to consider the influence of the whole body, approaching voice in a holistic way rather than just attending to the sound in isolation.

The head is balanced on the top of the spine, which is a flexible bony column that gives support to the trunk of the body. It is made up of 24 small bones called vertebrae; the top seven in the neck are called cervical vertebrae and it is the first of these, the atlas, that supports the skull. Below the neck are the 12 thoracic vertebrae (to which the ribs are attached) and five lumbar vertebrae. Discs of cartilage separate the ring-shaped vertebrae. At the lower end of the spine is the pelvis, the bony structure that connects the spine with the legs, consisting of the hip bones on each side and the sacrum and coccyx behind. The bones of the pelvis protect the soft abdominal organs within them and, of course, support the base of the spine. The interrelationship of head, spine, pelvis and ribcage is, as has been said, critically important for efficient and effective voicing to occur.

What is voice?

So, what is 'voice'? Where does it come from and what is the process that changes silent thought into spoken word? Two absolute requirements for the production of sound of any kind are a source of energy and a vibrating structure. The primary source of energy for voice production is a smooth flow of air provided by the lungs which the vibrating vocal folds convert into sound. Although the vocal folds are the principal source of sound, it is possible to constrict the vocal tract elsewhere along its length and create fricative noise, e.g. /s/ or /sh/, or indeed a temporary blocking of the flow of air through the vocal tract followed by a sudden release of the air pressure can produce a mildly explosive sound, e.g. /p/ and /t/. In continuous speech both voiced (sounds produced at the level of the larynx) and unvoiced sounds are produced. An analogue of the speech mechanism would have: a power supply – breath; a vibrating element – the vocal folds; a system of valves – the vocal tract; and a filtering device – the resonators.

Energy in the form of air from the lungs passes into the trachea and the larynx. The larynx is the principal structure for producing a vibrating airstream and the vocal folds, which are part of the larynx, make up the vibrating elements. The vocal folds are long, smoothly rounded bands of muscle tissue which may be lengthened, shortened, tensed and relaxed, as well as opened and closed across the airway. During normal breathing they are wide apart, the airstream is unimpeded, and air flows in and out of the lungs in regular phases. For speech, however, the vocal folds are closed or adducted, to restrict the flow of air from the lungs, while at the same time air pressure below the folds increases and the vocal folds are literally blown apart, releasing a puff of air into the vocal tract. This release of air results in a decrease in pressure below the folds and the elasticity of the tissue, plus the reduction of air pressure, allows them to snap back into their closed position ready to begin this cycle of vocal fold vibration again. In normal vowel production such vibrations occur at a rate of about 135 complete vibrations per second for men, about 235 vibrations per second for women and even more for children. This periodic interrupting of the airstream produces a vocal tone that is amplified within the pharyngeal, oral and nasal cavities, and transformed through articulation of the lips, tongue and teeth, resulting in meaningful speech sounds.

It can be seen from this brief description that, for sustained speech, good breath support, plenty of air, and flexible and relaxed respiratory muscles are needed, as are healthy and flexible vocal folds and free use of the resonators. Looking at each system in a little more detail, three quite separate but interconnecting systems emerge.

The respiratory system

The main purpose of the respiratory system is to maintain life by carrying air into the lungs, where the exchange of the gases oxygen and carbon dioxide takes place. The respiratory system begins at the nose and mouth and ends with the alveoli in the lungs. The nasal and oral cavities (the nose and mouth) and the pharynx and larynx are known collectively as the upper respiratory tract, whereas the lower respiratory tract refers to the trachea, the bronchi and the lungs, which are housed within the bony thoracic or chest cavity. In addition to its role in respiration the upper respiratory tract functions in the processes of swallowing, chewing, articulation, resonance and phonation, whereas the lower respiratory tract functions exclusively for the processes of breathing for life support and for the production of speech.

The respiratory tract, as has been noted, has two parallel entrances – the nose and the mouth – through which air enters. These merge into a common tract or pharynx. The area within the pharynx immediately behind the nose (called the nasopharynx) and the area behind the mouth (called the oropharynx) are separated by a muscular valve, the soft palate, which when raised can close off one section from another, so that, when we swallow, food and liquid do not escape through the nose. In the production of nasal consonants /n/, /m/ and /ng/ the soft palate is lowered to allow these sounds to be resonated in the nose.

The respiratory tract continues, passing through the larynx and the open vocal folds into the trachea. The trachea divides into two branches: into the smaller bronchi that enter the lungs and ultimately into the even smaller alveoli. The pear-shaped lungs are contained within the bony ribcage, consisting of 12 pairs of ribs. The first pair of ribs is immobile, attached at the front to the sternum or breastbone and at the back to the spinal vertebrae. Pairs two to seven are similarly attached, but by synovial joints which permit a degree of rotation, whereas pairs eight to ten are attached to each other at the front by flexible cartilage and pairs eleven and twelve (sometimes referred to as 'floating ribs') are fixed at the back to the spinal vertebrae, but have no fixed attachment at the front. This arrangement of the ribs is important, because, as the lungs are contained within this bony cage and linked to it by pleural and membranous tissue, alterations in the size and shape of the lungs when breathing in and out can be accommodated. This expansion is limited to the base of the lungs, because the tops of the lungs are constrained by the fixed immobile ribs at the top of the ribcage.

When we breathe in, the lungs expand and, to accommodate their increase in size, the diaphragm (a large dome-shaped muscle which separates the cavity of the chest from that of the abdomen) contracts, so increasing the vertical space within the ribcage. At the same time there is an increase in the width of the chest from front to back as a result of the movement of the upper ribs, which moves the sternum upwards and forwards. The link that exists between the lungs and the ribcage means that expansion or contraction of the lungs, when breathing in or out, will be mirrored by changes in the ribcage which will be either raised or lowered respectively, as a result of the movements of the intercostal muscles. For quiet respiration these changes are rarely noticed, the movement is so limited. It is only when additional air is taken in to support speech or song that the increased movement of the ribcage may be readily identified.

It is essential that the respiratory muscles are as flexible and efficient as possible in order to achieve this movement of the ribcage. The greater the expansion of the thoracic cavity, the greater the volume of air that can be contained within the lungs and, in order to achieve this, the individual must rely on muscular flexibility and support.

There is a difference between quiet, at-rest 'breathing for life', which relies on equal phases of inspiration and expiration, and modified inspiration for the purposes of speech and song, where a quick intake and slow release of air are essential, with the latter requiring much more active muscular control over respiration. The main respiratory muscles are listed here and illustrated in Figures 4.1 and 4.2. It should be noted that their effectiveness in supporting breath is very much affected by posture and tension.

Muscles of inspiration

These muscles are responsible for raising the ribcage and increasing the thoracic volume:

- The diaphragm: this large dome-shaped involuntary muscle is of great importance in respiration, playing the chief part in filling the lungs.

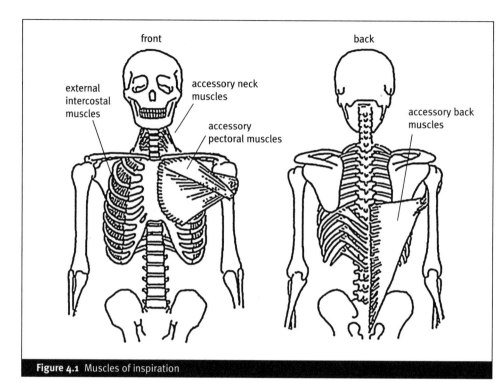

Figure 4.1 Muscles of inspiration

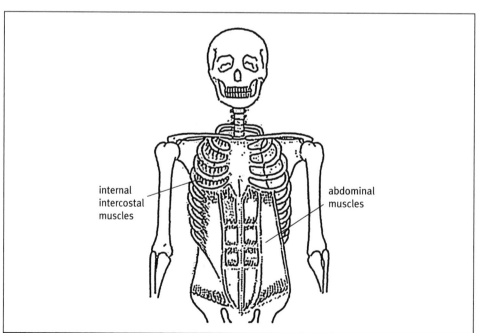

Figure 4.2 Muscles of expiration

During sleep and unconsciousness it maintains respiration under involuntary control.

- External intercostal muscles act to control the amount of space between the ribs.
- Accessory neck muscles act to help in elevation of the first and second ribs during inspiration.
- Accessory back muscles contribute to rib movement during inspiration.
- Accessory pectoral muscles contribute to expansion of the upper ribcage.

Muscles of expiration

These muscles are responsible for lowering the ribcage and decreasing the thoracic volume:

- Abdominal muscles: responsible for a decrease in the dimensions of the thoracic cavity, helping air to flow out of the lungs.
- Back muscles act in aiding the ribs to depress.
- Internal intercostal muscles act to help control the amount of space between the ribs.

When looking at Figures 4.1 and 4.2, it is clear that for many their poor habitual posture will make it difficult to achieve optimum breath support and as a consequence the vocal folds will have much less support in terms of initiating and sustaining phonation. High shoulder posture, and back and neck tension will all affect smooth muscle movement and, for that reason, so many teachers find that one of the most critical first steps in achieving easier voicing is relaxation. Specific relaxation exercises may be found in Chapter 10.

The phonatory system

This is the system that produces the sound known as voice. It consists of the larynx, or as it is more generally referred to 'the voice box', its muscles and ligaments, and the hyoid bone, from which the larynx is suspended and to which several extrinsic laryngeal muscles are attached. Continuous with the trachea below and the pharynx above, the principal biological function of the larynx is to act as a valve. This valve prevents air from escaping from the lungs, prevents foreign substances from entering the larynx and expels foreign substances that bypass the epiglottis and threaten to enter the trachea.

Situated in the neck at the level of the third to sixth cervical vertebrae, the larynx extends from the base of the tongue to the trachea. Not a single structure, the larynx is very small indeed, only 5 cm long in total and made up of nine individual cartilages: three large single cartilages, the thyroid, cricoid and epiglottis, and three paired cartilages, the arytenoid, corniculate and cuneiform (Figure 4.3).

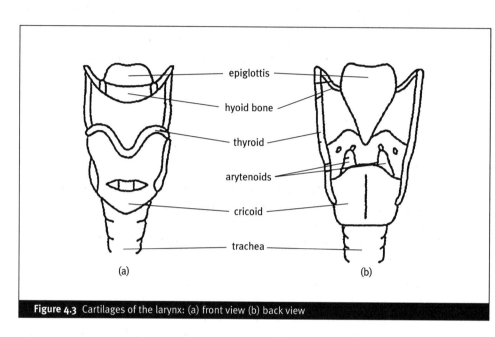

(a)   (b)

Figure 4.3 Cartilages of the larynx: (a) front view (b) back view

The principal cartilages of the larynx are as follows.

The epiglottis

This is a broad leaf-shaped cartilage, which is attached to the thyroid cartilage and projects upwards towards the tongue. The epiglottis changes position with tongue movements, and alters the size and shape of the pharyngeal cavity.

The thyroid cartilage

This is the biggest cartilage, shaped like a shield, which forms most of the front and side walls of the larynx. It is composed of four quadrilateral plates fused at the front and this junction or angle of the thyroid is most visible in men and commonly called the 'Adam's apple'. The vocal folds extend from the inside of the thyroid angle to the arytenoid cartilages.

The cricoid cartilage

This cartilage is just below the thyroid cartilage and immediately above the trachea and attached to the thyroid cartilage by the cricotracheal ligament. Shaped like a signet ring it is narrow in front and broad behind, and forms the base of the larynx.

Arytenoid cartilages

These small pyramid-shaped cartilages articulate with the cricoid cartilage via the cricoarytenoid joints. The arytenoids are the vocal gymnasts; they can in fact glide medially and laterally and rotate slightly, and may also slide forwards and backwards but with restricted movement. Almost any combination of the above can occur simultaneously. Their importance in the production of voice lies in the fact that the vocal folds have an attachment to these cartilages via the vocal process so that the specialized nature of their movements is essential in allowing the vocal folds to open and close with ease and thus produce changes in pitch (Figure 4.4).

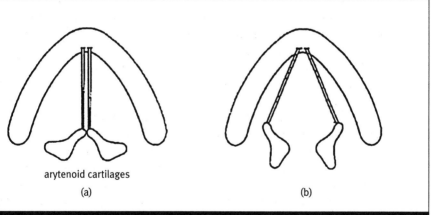

arytenoid cartilages

(a)

(b)

Figure 4.4 Schematic illustration of the movement of the arytenoid cartilages and consequent movement of the vocal cords: (a) closure (b) opening

The vocal folds

The paired thyroarytenoid muscles make up the body of the vocal fold. The thyroarytenoid muscle has a superior portion, which forms the false vocal fold (mainly concerned with making a firm seal when swallowing occurs) and an inferior portion, which forms the true vocal fold. In contrast to the red false folds, the true vocal folds are white in colour. In men the vocal folds are between 17 and 23 mm in length, with those of women slightly shorter at approximately 12–17 mm long. The space between the false and true vocal folds is known as the laryngeal ventricle and is well supplied with mucous glands, thereby lubricating the vocal folds and protecting them in part from the effects of friction. Within the larynx and the vocal tract, the mucous membrane is usually moist, but dryness of the membranous cover of the vocal folds, caused by infection, smoke and the physiological effects of stress, will noticeably affect the voice. The very specialized structure of the vocal folds, composed of four different tissue layers, each with different mechanical properties important for vibration, accounts for the amazing range and versatility of the voice.

The resonatory system

The resonatory system consists of the chest and the pharyngeal, oral and nasal cavities. The resonators above the larynx can alter in size, shape and tension through movement of the base of the tongue and the soft palate. In addition further modification can occur through contraction of the pharyngeal and extrinsic laryngeal muscles. Although the larynx is obviously the primary contributor to the production of voice, without the acoustic influence of the resonators, the voice would sound very thin indeed. Most of the quality and loudness characteristics that are associated with the voice are the result of the resonators. In the same way that the weak vibrations of the strings of a musical instrument are altered by the resonating body of the instrument, so the tone that is produced at the level of the larynx, the laryngeal buzz, is altered by the resonators. The airway above the larynx acts like an acoustic filter, which can suppress or maximize some sounds as they pass through. Alterations can also occur in the configuration of the vocal tract by varying tongue positions, raising or lowering the soft palate, and as an effect of the degree of relaxation or tension present. For the skilled professional voice user, the effective use of the resonators can be a powerful tool in increasing the range and power of the voice, e.g. contrast the open mouth position adopted by singers and actors with the sound heard from speakers with limited mouth opening. Exercises in Chapter 10 include suggestions for working on resonance.

Hormonal changes

The specialized structure of the vocal folds is, as with the rest of the body, influenced by hormonal (endocrinological) and ageing changes. Hormonal changes account for the voice breaks and uncertain pitch that occur in the male voice at puberty, where the vocal folds increase in length and thickness. For women, hormonal changes at puberty, during menstruation and pregnancy cause an increase in fluid retention, resulting in an increase in vocal fold mass, or 'swelling' of the vocal folds. This, in turn, leads to a temporary lowering of the speaking fundamental frequency of the voice, with a subsequent change in vocal quality. As with any musical instrument, if the free edges of the vocal folds are damaged, swollen, dry or lacking in tension, the resultant sound will be less than adequate. Typically, swollen vocal folds will give a husky, harsh, breathy quality; the free edges do not meet cleanly to vibrate easily together as a result of the increased mass or swelling, and often air escapes leading to the breathy sound. It should, however, be noted that in many cases the changes are very subtle and may be perceived by only either a professional voice user or an experienced voice professional.

Professional singers may stipulate a clause in their contracts to allow them to withdraw from performances in the premenstrual phase of the cycle. Mathieson (2001) notes that singers report a range of vocal changes related to the premenstrual phase, specifically problems of pitch range, vocal quality and unpredictability of vocal function. Women who are using their voices extensively with heavy vocal loading should be particularly aware that their voices might be vulnerable at this time.

The menopause signals a reduction of ovarian hormones and this decrease in oestrogen levels again leads to an increase in vocal fold mass, although instead of this effecting a temporary change in pitch, as in the premenstrual period, the change in postmenopausal pitch is permanent. In addition to perceptual voice quality changes such as reduction in pitch, and a narrow register, other changes such as lack of vocal intensity, vocal fatigue, decreased lubrication of the vocal folds, increased rigidity, decreased flexibility and rigidity of the cricothryroid all occur. For some women, however, androgens, which contribute to a loss of secretion, become oestrogen in fat cells, thereby indirectly reversing some of the vocal effects of postmenopausal loss of oestrogen in those women with greater stores of fat cells. It should also be remembered that female hormonal changes do not occur in isolation; significant age-related changes will be occurring throughout the body at the same time and the effect of these changes on the vocal process should not be underestimated.

Effects of ageing

Changes in pitch level and pitch range in boys' voices, which accompany pubertal change, are well recognized. By age 15, Hirano et al. (1983) suggest that full vocal ligaments have been developed by both males and females, but the female larynx shows much less dramatic change at puberty than that of the male; although changes in girls' voices also occur, they are less well recognized.

Changes in pitch range are noted as individuals enter 'middle' age. Again differences between male and female voices are noted, specifically at the age at which these changes occur. Ageing changes in the male larynx tend to occur in the fourth decade; for women, as has already been noted, these changes occur at the time of the menopause, usually in the fifth decade. These changes are the result of specific tissue structural changes that occur within the folds, so that the cover undergoes alteration; epithelial thickening is observed (i.e. changes occur in the upper cellular layer of the vocal fold) and changes in the underlying connective tissue result in looser linkage of the epithelium to the deeper tissues. The elastic fibres of the vocal ligaments break down and become thinner whereas the mucous glands degenerate, resulting in less adequate lubrication of the vocal fold surface and probable changes in the biomechanical properties of the superficial epithelium. As with other muscles, the laryngeal muscles are prone to atrophy, which means that there are fewer muscle fibres in each muscle and in addition the surviving fibres tend to be thinner and to show significant degenerative changes. It is possible that these changes result from disturbances of the blood supply.

As the vocal folds become less elastic, bowing can occur; the vocal folds cannot vibrate along their full length, leading to a weak breathy note. This seems to be particularly a problem with older men, leading to a thinner higher voice, whereas women, as we have said, tend to have slightly thicker more swollen vocal folds in older age, limiting their range. In addition there would appear to be a trend towards a decrease in range with increasing age. Laryngeal cartilages calcify, a process that begins quite early in adulthood and starts sooner and is more complete in men than in women.

By old age the changes are quite extensive in both sexes and certainly the vocal folds of old people look very different from those of younger adults. There is frequently greyish or yellowish discoloration of the tissue, loss of mass and a residual gap on vocal fold closure.

As well as changes within the larynx, ageing brings about changes within the lungs, which deteriorate with increasing age; of course smoking accelerates this deterioration. Reduction of the mobility of the thoracic cage occurs, the ribs become less mobile and, with advanced age, the lungs and bronchi shrink and sink to a lower position in the thorax, although the sensitivity of the airway is reduced and coughing is less likely to occur. Physical activity will prevent noticeable deterioration in respiration and it is important to avoid pollutants, because these will affect the elastic recoil of the lungs. With declining respiratory function, voice quality is affected as a result of lack of breath support. If, however, attention is paid to postural, respiratory and vocal health, it is possible to maintain a voice that sounds much younger than an individual's chronological age.

There are, therefore, changes in the sound of the voice and alterations to the larynx that accompany ageing, although it would be inappropriate to suggest that all the changes are the result of alterations to the laryngeal cartilages. Indeed, it may be that the loss of flexibility within the vocal folds means that glottal closure becomes less complete and less stable, and results in a sound that is perceived as being somewhat rough and perhaps breathy. This quality is one that is associated with older individuals.

5 Voice as a physical skill

When the voice is used to communicate, it is not just the larynx and the organs of speech that are involved in the process, but the whole body. Chapter 4 highlighted the many muscles used in the production of sound. In addition to these muscles, the spine and the relationship of the pelvis, ribcage, head, neck and shoulder girdle to the spine have a significant effect on the voice.

This sense of the physicality of voice is not always recognized, partly because the significance of this link has not always been well defined and partly because an accurate sense of physical self is not generally well developed. Asked, for example, to close his or her eyes and, using the hands, indicate the width of his or her hips, head or waist, or the length of the foot, an individual will generally overestimate the size. There is also often a mistaken assumption by individuals that they are taller or shorter than they actually are, even when judging height in comparison with other people whom they know well. Some individuals have little concept of themselves within space; they duck unnecessarily when passing through doorways and, when asked to explore the space behind themselves, agree that this is an area that they do not generally consider that they inhabit. There is a tendency for the same spatial levels to be used repeatedly. In an effort to reconfigure personal space, the following exercise is very effective: imagine being in a personal glass sphere and use hands and feet to touch and explore the outer limits of it, and in this way open up a 'new' special dimension. We associate voice quality with hearing rather than feeling. It is useful to begin to think of the voice as vibration, which may be felt as well as heard.

Vocal culture

It is said that society in the late twentieth and early twenty-first centuries has become very cerebral, with individuals 'living' in their heads. Language has become a means of expressing ideas and conveying information in contrast to the physical and emotional language of what are sometimes described pejoratively as 'less sophisticated' societies, whose cultures are more vocally liberated and who have maintained a strong tradition of song, dance and story-telling in their communities. Loud voices accompanied by expansive physical gestures tend to be considered flamboyant or excessive in certain western countries. Lack of voice/body connection, combined with a lack of understanding of the link between body and voice, can limit an individual's ability to recognize the early warning signs of a voice in trouble.

Body balance

Many vocal problems are the indirect result of a lack of balance in body alignment. This balance can be altered by a serious event such as a back injury or fracture of the ribs, where an individual can unconsciously restrict movement in that part of the body to avoid discomfort. Similarly foot, back, neck, shoulder or chest pain can restrict movement and alter posture. Even something as simple as a change of footwear – a change in the heel height of a pair of shoes – can tip the natural balance of the pelvis, and thereby affect spine, head and shoulder alignment with a consequent effect on the voice.

The spine

The spine reaches from the head to the coccyx. It is made up of the vertebrae, between each of which are intervertebral discs, cartilages that separate one vertebra from another and provide a cushion. The spine has a certain amount of flexibility and it also has natural curves. The flexibility of the spine and its curves allows a range of movement to be undertaken without injury – the curves in the spine absorbing, for example, the shock of jolting and landing when jumping. The spine, most importantly, shields the spinal cord and the nerve fibres come through the openings between the vertebrae. Often, the term 'straighten the spine' is used when correcting alignment, but it is important to retain the spinal curves and, without over-exaggerating or straightening them, for the spine to feel long. Figure 5.1 shows the necessary curves in the neck, thoracic and lumbar regions of the spine.

When the spine loses its natural length as a result of factors associated with illness or ageing, it is important to note that the ribcage, which is attached to the spine and houses the lungs, becomes depressed. This usually results in the slumping forward of the shoulders so that the entire 'front' of the body closes downwards and inwards. Space for breathing to

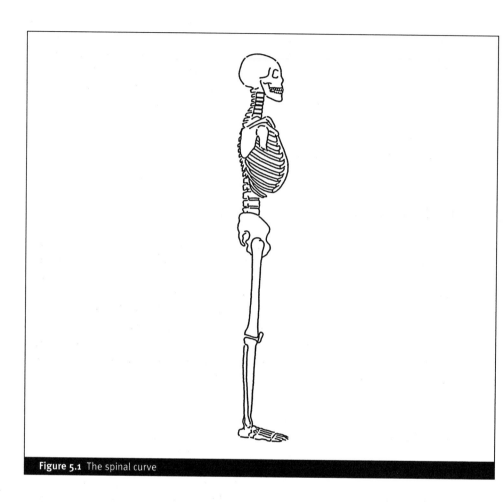

Figure 5.1 The spinal curve

occur easily, as well as the elasticity of the ribs, is therefore lost. At the top of the spine is the head, positioned on what is called the atlanto-occipital joint, the joint between the top vertebra and the bottom of the skull.

The head

Asking participants in workshops how much they think the head weighs encourages a range of responses, from the very light, 2 or 3 pounds, a little over a kilogram, to the much more accurate 12–15 pounds, or 6 kg. 'Guessing the weight of the head' has a serious intent, aiming both to impress on individuals the effort required to achieve a critical balance between the head, considering its heavy weight, and the neck and spine, and to consider what the implications of this are for the voice.

If an item of similar weight were to be carried comfortably, it would, quite naturally, be held close to the body rather than at arm's length. Consider then the tension created when the neck is extended forward and the head, as a consequence, rather than being balanced easily on top of the spine, is similarly extended so that critical head/neck alignment is lost. The effect of this is to recruit the large muscles of the neck, jaw and shoulders in order to compensate for this loss of alignment. The effect of this compensatory action is far reaching because, as has already been noted, there is a direct link between these muscles and the larynx. Proper alignment allows the body to move effectively and harmoniously, without creating unnecessary tensions.

To illustrate this more effectively the following exercise is recommended: two individuals 'pair' off; one of the pair lies on the floor and the other sits at his or her head, gently easing any tension in the prone individual's shoulder area by massaging. Before the next stage, which is carefully to take the weight of the other's head in the hands, it is important to reassure the 'prone' individual that the head will not be handled roughly or let drop to the floor after being lifted. To begin with the head usually feels very light because the individual on the floor is using the large muscles of the neck to hold the weight. Once he or she trusts the 'holder' enough the person may gradually give up control and when this happens the holder will begin to experience the true weight of the head and find that it is possible to move the head gently from side to side without interference from the 'owner'.

Practical suggestions

An easy way for individuals working on their own to experience the weight of the head is to lie on the floor and lift the head about an inch off the ground. Feeling the stress that this places on the muscles of the neck gives an idea of the benefits of balancing the head on the top of the spine in an effortless manner, leaving all the muscles of the neck, jaw and shoulders stress free. It will also allow the jaw to move freely, not restricting the movement needed to produce voice and speech.

An excellent exercise for developing awareness in the top of the neck is that of the 'nodding dog' or 'marionette'. This exercise involves isolating the small muscles that allow the head to rock gently in a smooth, weightless manner, rather like the movement of the toy dogs found on car dash-boards that have a head attached to the body by a large spring. As the car moves the head wobbles – a very similar movement is seen on the puppets in films of the *Thunderbirds*.

1. To practise the exercise, which can be done sitting or standing, it is important first to feel length in the neck and then to exercise the large muscles by drawing imaginary floor-to-ceiling lines with the nose. Start these lines at the right shoulder and move across to the left 'using' the nose as a pen. This exercise allows the uppermost neck muscles, which contract in stress, to stretch and release.
2. Still using the nose as a pen draw a fluid figure of eight, firstly in the normal upright manner and then as if it were lying on its side, so moving across to the right side and then through the centre point to the left side.
3. Imagine a column of water is spouting up the spine and the head is floating on the top of it. Feel the weightlessness of the head.
4. Allow the head to bounce gently on the spine like a marionette. Make all moves in slow motion first.
5. Making sure that the jaw is not clenched, try gentle 'yes' nods, then 'no' nods and finally try to use both in a 'nodding dog' movement. These take some practice but they give a very useful awareness to the area of the body most involved in the 'fight-or-flee' positions.

Unlocking the knees

An area of the body that is not immediately associated with voice is the knee area. Most individuals brace their knees in order to steady themselves, particularly when they are under stress. Individuals unused to the

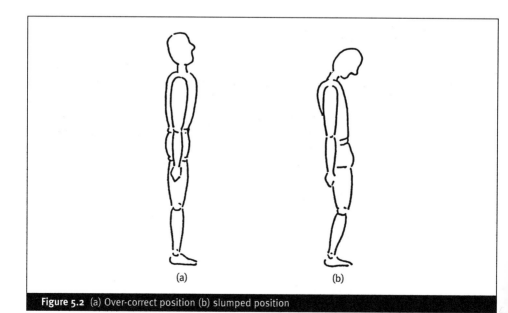

Figure 5.2 (a) Over-correct position (b) slumped position

experience of public speaking or performing, often remark 'My knees were shaking' or 'I went weak at the knees'. When the knees are locked, a lower abdominal tension is created which interferes with diaphragmatic movement. For the breath to flow in and out of the body, it is important to stand in a balanced and open manner, with the knees released and flexed, the feet in contact with the floor, and the body arranged around the spine with the feeling that it is lengthened and wide.

The term 'lengthen' is often used in connection with posture. This comes from the Alexander Technique which teaches the need gently to oppose the force of gravity that seems intent on 'squashing' us downward and inward. The word 'oppose' is preferable to 'fight' because it does not bring with it images of over-correction. It is as common to find over-corrected, regimented posture as it is to find slumped, contracted posture; what is less common is the open, lengthened and wide 'ideal'.

It could be said that an individual's habitual posture is a measure of the way in which he or she responds to and handles the stress of daily living. Similarly, for many teachers their posture reflects the stresses of contemporary teaching. Some seem bowed by the volume of work and the seemingly insurmountable pressures; others take on the 'struggle' – literally – with chin thrust forwards and shoulders braced (Figure 5.2).

The importance of eye level

The physical effect that eye level has on the body and therefore the voice is often under-estimated. Shy children and socially intimidated, or depressed, individuals often avoid eye contact and adopt a lowered head position. This has a domino effect: the sternum becomes depressed, resulting in a lack of openness in the ribs and pressure on the abdomen. As a consequence the individual is unable to achieve more than a very shallow breath, which in turn produces a monotonous vocal quality. The opposite of this is a rigidly fixed focus which tends to correspond to locked neck, clenched jaw and stiffly held shoulders, leading to an enormous amount of unuseful tension. This posture limits peripheral vision, because the eyes do not scan, but look fixedly ahead, giving an impression of aggression and rigidity. Tension limits the free exchange of breath and results in a vocal quality that is often strident, lacks flexibility and warmth, and can appear aggressive.

Open and balanced alignment encourages peripheral vision, and the individual is able to function within their world in an aware and integrated manner. These rather 'extreme' examples are included to signal the importance of posture not only in determining vocal quality but also in how an individual is perceived by others.

The child's ability to shout

Most primary school children in the playground are able to scream and shout during play time without losing their voices. There are a number of reasons for this: first, they tend to have natural alignment; second, they are playing so that their activities are free of harmful negative tensions (although no one would deny the positive tension involved in exuberant play); and, third, they are generally using the whole chest and *releasing* the outgoing breath rather than *holding* it. There are, of course, exceptions to these generalizations; some children develop nodules or polyps on the vocal folds through improper use (Hunt and Slater, 2003) but they remain, fortunately, a minority of the school-age population.

Secondary school children present a very different picture. There is a considerable difference between the open and proud posture of the average 6 year old and that of the average 16 year old. When teachers in workshops are asked to demonstrate the posture of children in the class, boys are portrayed very differently from girls. When representing male posture, two very different stereotypical postures are portrayed: either the assumed confidence of the tight high-shouldered swagger, or a slumped spine body position with a concave chest, low eye level, with the head bowed in front of the shoulders. Girls are often portrayed as slumping forward with arms folded across the chest, or in some cases around the waist. In both boys and girls the significant similarity is the weight distribution, which is usually across one foot or hip, not two, resulting in a loss of space between the lower ribs and the hips, limiting the ribs' ability to widen and increase breath capacity and support the voice through expansion of the lower lung area.

Changes in adolescence

Just why this change from easy open posture and alignment to tight, contracted or slumped stance occurs in the adolescent, and in some cases the pre-adolescent, years is a subject open to much discussion. It is obviously the result of a number of factors. As children grow, particularly if they have a sudden 'growth spurt', they may temporarily lose some motor control and can appear ungainly, e.g. they may walk into objects or stub their toes. The way that they feel about themselves and their developing bodies can make them feel vulnerable and exposed. Much of the body language seen is an attempt either to protect themselves by withdrawing from society and making themselves inconspicuous by occupying as little space as possible, or to assume a confidence that they do not feel by lifting the shoulders, thrusting the jaw and taking up a greater amount

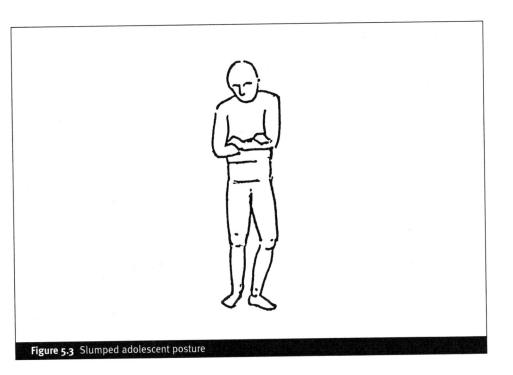

Figure 5.3 Slumped adolescent posture

of physical space. During this period, holding eye contact in everyday communication is extremely difficult because some young people cannot bring themselves to confront adults, so their eye level tends to be lowered and this produces the head/neck alignment that develops a slumped spine and results in shallow breathing (Figure 5.3).

In some teenagers it is possible to see the development of the use of head, neck and jaw in conveying the body language of either aggression or fear. The threatening body language of the forward thrust jaw or the low eye levels found in the fearful and insecure is familiar. These ancillary movements of the neck, shoulder and head in response to fear and anger are artefacts of the 'fight-or-flee' response, also referred to as the 'startle' effect by teachers of the Alexander Technique.

Language has assimilated similar attitudes to voice and body language. Sayings such as 'be brave, take it on the chin', 'keep your chin up', 'you look as if you are carrying the world on your shoulders' are familiar, as is 'take a deep breath' or 'grin and bear it' in difficult situations when courage is needed. In situations that promote frustration, 'being lost for words' or 'speechless' or 'being so angry I could not speak' or, in cases of sadness, the phrase 'having a lump in my throat' is familiar. Reticent speakers are often referred to as 'tongue tied', whereas the loquacious have 'the gift of the gab'.

Adulthood

Adults seldom correct or change the habits of adolescence; postural and movement patterns have been set and these continue to provide a pattern for adult life. Even when trying to absorb new patterns of alignment, the body 'prefers' the old pattern, often rejecting the new posture as 'wrong' because it identifies and is comfortable with its habitual posture. For this reason, should posture be suspected to be a contributing factor in a voice problem, it is a very good idea to seek advice and to work with the help of an 'outside eye'. There are many people who can help, from physiotherapists, osteopaths, Alexander Technique and Feldenkrais teachers, to Qi Gong, Tai Chi and yoga teachers.

It is important to find someone who is qualified to work with the body therapeutically; practical help and advice need to be directed towards recognizing the uniqueness of each individual and fulfilling individual needs. For this reason, the advice on alignment offers general principles but working with a teacher in a 'hands-on' manner is strongly advised, if possible. If, however, there is no alternative to working alone, some of the following suggestions may be useful.

Some useful physical strategies

Video

Posture, as has been noted above, is difficult to change because, in spite of the fact that it may need correction, it is habitual and therefore natural and comfortable. It is very difficult for individuals to 'step outside themselves', to see themselves as others see them. A mirror although useful does not offer the profile or back view, but an excellent alternative is to use a video to record movement and habitual posture. Video provides accurate feedback for those who need to work on posture but do not really understand what adjustments need to be made. A video recording made when the individual concerned is not conscious of the camera is a particularly useful tool. It is important to view the video with objectivity, rather than with a degree of vanity or too critically, noting the head/shoulder relationship and the natural but unexaggerated curves in the lower back and thoracic spine. Notice also whether the head is carried forward or correctly balanced on the top of the spine. This exercise is best undertaken individually or in very small groups who are happy to take suggestions from each other. It is important not simply to force the body into a new posture, but to use the information gleaned from the video to build a sense of physical awareness.

Spot reminders

A very successful way of re-patterning the physical memory is to use the simple method of applying small coloured spots to strategic points around the home, office or classroom, e.g. as a reminder to relax the shoulders, a spot placed on the wall near the telephone in easy view will act as a trigger when speaking on the phone, to encourage the individual to check shoulder position.

Holding the phone between shoulder and head, while the hands are involved in other activities such as looking up references, cooking or writing, can affect vocal quality. Other useful positions for spots are on the fridge door, or the edge of a VDU or typewriter, on the steering wheel of the car, on the edge of the classroom blackboard or on the school piano.

Alignment

Many industrial and commercial businesses are investing in postural training because of the number of working days lost through back injury and issues related to Health and Safety regulations. Similar training in school or college provided by a physiotherapist, osteopath, Alexander teacher or similar physical therapist is strongly recommended.

Effort levels

When stress levels are high, it is more difficult than usual to assess effort levels, a task that is not easy even when most relaxed. Effort levels are usually assessed as either high or low depending on intrinsic and extrinsic mood and demand levels. It is, however, useful to be able to gauge physical and vocal effort levels so that energy may be expended appropriately and not wasted unnecessarily – stress is tiring and unproductive. The efficient use of energy and effort depends on developing awareness of the degrees of effort necessary for specific tasks and matching the effort to the demand.

Suggested exercise

An easy exercise to help to familiarize individuals with their own effort levels is to shake hands in pairs. Person A asks person B to shake hands and then to rate his or her own handshake on an effort scale of 1–10. If, for example, they rate it at 7, A then asks B to shake at effort level 3 or 9, then return to 7, go down to 4, and so on, until he or she has established a graduated scale of effort. The partners then change over and repeat the exercise.

This exercise has a practical application for voice use. Start by sounding a well-supported /ah/ vowel with varying degrees of energy, moving up the scale from 1 to 10 and assessing the different vocal effort needed for each stage. In this way the individual will begin to have a more accurate understanding of the amount of vocal effort, either high or low, that is consistent with specific vocal demands. Once this is achieved, and the level of vocal energy is spontaneously allied to the effort level, the exercise can be extended to short familiar classroom phrases or instruction, e.g. 'put your books away now', or 'line up quietly class 4'.

6 Communication

Professional voice users, the group to which teachers and lecturers belong, are, in the jargon of the day, in the 'communication business', but sometimes the skills of 'getting the message across' either have never been learned or else have been given a low priority. This is, perhaps, not surprising in the face of the current teacher workload and, indeed, the heavy academic pressures that teachers have to face before qualifying. It is, however, one of the most essential skills for a teacher; how often is a teacher remembered, not for the content of the lesson but for the enthusiasm and energy that he or she brought to the lesson? Often this influenced his or her pupils' or students' future subject choice and even future career choices. It is perhaps salutary to think of how few teachers in school life are remembered as having had this ability to share their enthusiasm for their subject with their pupils and students and really to communicate. Most teachers are enthusiastic about their subject, but some are unable to share that enthusiasm because their communication skills are limited. This chapter suggests some aspects of communication and self-presentation skills that teachers might find of benefit.

What exactly is meant by communication? The process of communication can be divided broadly into two areas: verbal and non-verbal. Verbal communication is generally thought of solely as speech but speech as it is perceived is composed of several interdependent elements, which are outlined below.

Language

The ability to convert ideas into words is fundamental to the communication process. There is no point in having the most wonderful appreciation of a subject without an ability to find words with which to transmit these ideas fluently and imaginatively to others, and in a form relevant to the audience. Effective speech is the process of getting an idea from one mind to another, accurately and persuasively. There are few people who have attended lectures and not experienced the 'woolly talker' –

those individuals who know exactly what they mean, but are the only ones in the room who do.

This is where the choice of words, their arrangement and the way in which they are expressed are the tools that will achieve this end most effectively. Language lives, changes and responds to different social and cultural mores, and the fact that the English language has the capacity to change and to grow creatively, by absorbing vocabulary from other cultures and countries, has made it the dynamic language that it is today. In France, where the use of grammatically correct spoken and written language is intimately connected to nationalist identity, there was an attempt in 1995 to ban certain foreign words, mainly English and American, from advertisements and public pronouncements. The attempt was ill-conceived and subjected to a certain amount of ridicule. English has always had the capacity to take and make its own vocabulary from elsewhere. This is what allows language to grow and survive in a truly pragmatic way.

So the choice of words will convey, more or less effectively, the meaning to the listener but the way in which the words are expressed will affect the impact that the message has on the listener. Within the area of verbal communication other parameters of speech need to be considered, namely, articulation, voice quality and vocal variety, which underpin the way that words are expressed.

Articulation

Articulation is the way in which speech sounds are produced in order to make language intelligible to the listener. The clarity of speech depends on the accuracy of the movements of the articulators: tongue, lips, jaw and teeth. The current vogue for a lack of precise articulation often leads to a loss of understanding; if what the speaker is saying is not completely understood there is a tendency for the listener to 'switch off'. Positioning plays an important role in aiding understanding because it is often particularly difficult for pupils when a teacher, whose articulation is not very precise, stands with his or her back to the class, writing notes on the whiteboard and giving information at the same time. The amount of reliance on lip-reading both to help and to confirm understanding is not always recognized. If a speaker cannot be seen, there is often a sense that the listener needs to listen harder.

To gain some appreciation of this, it is a useful exercise deliberately to look away from a speaker and judge how much added listening effort is needed to understand him or her, when facial expression, body posture and articulatory movements cannot be relied on to help.

There would appear to be a general perception that clear, precise articulation is somewhat outdated and decidedly unfashionable, and little value is currently placed on defined articulation. This is not to advocate a return to the rather clipped articulation of the 1940s and 1950s which black and white films so faithfully reproduce, but it is possible to be aware of articulation and to see it as a very useful tool in helping to maintain the class's interest. With clarity of articulation, there is less need for repetition and as a result there is less need to use the voice unnecessarily. The muscularity of speech is never fully present if the speaker is not mentally committed to the word; on the other hand, the enthusiastic teacher with a need to share ideas rarely has a problem being understood. Only when the synchronization of thought and word occurs is language wholly energized. A return to more energized use of consonants, particularly the explosive (voiced) consonants, /b/, /d/ and /g/ and (un-voiced) /p/, /t/ and /k/ brings a dynamic to language and produces the physical and vocal movement inherent in words such as bubble, hop, tap, bounce, kick, drag, slap and giggle.

Over-obvious manipulation of the dynamics of words is often seen as flamboyant, over-assertive or arrogant in our culture. Some individuals feel that they would be making themselves vulnerable by use of such 'overstated' voice or that they would appear pedantic. In truth it is possible to appear all these things if articulation is pushed or unrelated to the meaning behind it, but committed meaningful speech tends to engage the breath and muscles in the most positive way and produces naturally energized language.

There is something exciting about listening to an individual who is inspired by an idea. Watching children 'hang' on the words of an effective story-teller is to know the power that language has to access the imagination of the listener. The speech of young children is full of the sounds that they hear around them – 'splash', 'swoosh', 'ping', 'gurgle', the sounds of whistles, explosions and the noise of cars, motorbikes, aeroplanes and machinery. Of course those who read comics add the expletives such as 'Kapow!', 'Zap!' and 'Gadoom!' to their vocabulary, and when making these sounds they use the muscularity of speech in an uninhibited and joyous way. This playful use of the articulatory organs helps them to develop vocal and verbal muscle and imbue sound with energy that, regrettably, adults often lose. Practice, using carefully selected verse, can help to maintain the imaginative use of words, and adults too can explore their own use of language through prose and verse.

The use of the final consonant is essential in the delivery of any information and therefore critical in teaching. Conversational speech that is relaxed and delivered to one or two people does not require a deliberate weighting of consonants, but once the speech becomes public, that is to say to an audience or class, there is a need to form the consonants properly in order to aid definition and increase audibility, e.g. the final consonant in the word 'find' needs to be heard or the word could be confused with 'fine'. Male teachers should be aware that lip-reading is made more difficult by the addition of facial hair from beards or moustaches, so, for the more hirsute teacher, articulatory precision is even more important.

Voice

Voice works on many levels; first, it goes without saying, it makes speech audible, but it also gives definition to what is being said in many different ways, notably through changes in intonation and vocal pitch, alterations in pace, through the use of pause, by putting stress on particular syllables within words and by emphasizing certain words in sentences.

Other vocal parameters

For better identification of the discrete qualities of a number of other vocal parameters, they are examined separately in the following section.

Intonation

Intonation could be said to provide a vocal blueprint; it describes the way in which a specific voice alters during speech. The intonation pattern used, for example, when asking a question is very different from the one used to express an opinion. In a situation in which a speaker feels under-confident, a questioning vocal tune may be used because it seems to produce an impression of politeness and conciliation. This 'tune' can often be heard in the voices of teachers who work with pre-primary and infant schoolchildren, because it does not sound threatening or aggressive. When used inappropriately, however, it can give the impression of being uncertain and tentative. The other extreme is the continual use of the 'definite statement tune', which is often used by those in high status or authoritative positions, and generally used by newscasters, because it is perceived as being 'the truth' and not to be questioned. Although this is a confident and assertive tune, if used inappropriately it can make the listeners – pupils and students for example – feel that there is no space or opportunity for asking questions or sharing ideas.

Each language and dialect has an inherent 'tune' that expresses emotion and attitude. Even after a relatively short exposure to a language that is not their own, most individuals become aware of the 'tune' of the language. This then allows them, when listening to an exchange between speakers, to make an educated guess as to whether the speakers are having an argument, exchanging pleasantries or asking questions, just by the way in which the individual voices are moving through the pitch range.

The benefits of understanding the intricacies of human perceptions and assumptions are obvious, particularly as teachers and lecturers are continually interrelating with students and other members of staff on a verbal and vocal level. Particular emphasis should be given to this vocal parameter, when in an interview or an appraisal situation. More and more business and industrial courses are concentrating on the importance and power of paralinguistic skills. These are skills fundamental to the teacher's professional role, but ones that to date receive little attention during training.

Pitch

The pitch of the voice will often carry the emotional content of speech. When an individual becomes excited or stressed, vocal pitch often rises and the voice becomes shrill. In the same way, when frightened or very angry an individual may literally 'lose his or her voice', and be able only to whisper. Often individuals will use a very low vocal pitch when they are attempting to maintain control or when they are in a situation in which they want to appear more authoritative. Despite anti-sex discrimination legislation, in practical terms discrimination against women in the work place remains and is expressed covertly, if not overtly. One noted response to this phenomenon is the way in which many female executives, women in authority, teachers or women who are in competition with men have been advised to try consciously to adopt what could be called a gender-neutral vocal quality. This is not too high pitched and not too light in terms of resonance, yet not so deep as to appear masculine. The lower pitch is perceived as giving more status and, as a consequence, what they say will carry more weight. Under-pitching the voice, be it male or female, in this way, is not to be recommended, because it can often damage the voice and limit its range, resulting in an uninteresting, limited vocal quality.

Pace and rate

Alterations in pace, the speed at which an individual speaks, greatly influence the way in which the listener interprets what is being said. If excited and enthusiastic there is a tendency to speak more quickly. Think of individuals who speak very quickly – there is a sense of urgency behind what they are saying. This device can often be used in meetings where the fast talker virtually 'steam-rollers' the meeting; the rest of the group has no chance to interrupt and scarcely time to assimilate what is being said. At the opposite end of the spectrum, if uncertain about facts or simply unsure as to what position to take on a issue, an individual may slow speech down, become hesitant and frequently introduce fillers such as 'er' and 'um', appearing to weigh up each word. A consequence of this slow delivery is that the speaker may be perceived as demonstrating uncertainty, and this may encourage the listener to 'switch off' and disregard what is being said.

On the other hand a slow delivery may be seen as evidence of the speaker's commitment to an idea or an opinion and a sign of his or her confidence in expressing it. The advantage of using a fairly slow delivery rate is that it allows the speaker time to think ahead and make sure that he or she has complete control over what he or she is saying. Faster speech often does not allow the speaker to do this and spontaneous, or 'off the cuff', speech tends to be at a faster rate, although on occasions this may be the result of anxiety or stress and can result in gabbled speech. Politicians tend to use the device of slow speech, which allows them less chance of unwittingly blurting out an unreasoned opinion. To maintain the interest of the listener, however, it is important to allow the content to determine the pace of delivery, otherwise the predictability of pace becomes monotonous and unrelated to intention.

The vocal blueprint

Voice quality and vocal profile contribute in large measure to an individual's identity and the way in which he or she is perceived by others. Voice quality is very influential in the impressions that individuals give and receive. The visual picture represented by the disembodied voice of the radio announcer most easily demonstrates this. This representation is partly dependent on the sound of the voice – the vocal pitch, tone and quality of the resonance – partly on the accent of the speech and partly on the content and manner of delivery.

A number of research projects (Farb, 1973) have explored reactions to the 'disembodied voice' and found that listeners make a very definite assumption about the speaker. A similar process occurs when speaking to unfamiliar people on the phone; instinctive judgements are made about a range of attributes. These judgements can extend to the speaker's age, physical appearance, including height and weight, the educational background, family background and class, status, residential area, political persuasion, level of assertiveness and intelligence. Various subtle messages, conscious and unconscious, are conveyed by the tone of the voice and it is quite possible for the words to be 'saying' one thing and the voice to be 'saying' another. A cogent example of this is where, in response to asking someone how he or she is, the answer is 'fine', yet it is apparent that they are not fine. Feelings of low self-esteem, tension, tiredness, sadness or boredom are all reflected in the voice.

Vocal quality

There are certain vocal qualities that are perceived as more friendly than others; a speaker with warm 'mellow' tones seems to be interpreted as someone who can be trusted, who is sincere and friendly, whereas a 'harsher' more forced voice quality can appear aggressive and threatening. The voice plays an important role in the interview situation; the advantages for the individual candidate who is able to conceal nervousness by a relaxed vocal quality and the disadvantages for another who presents with a voice that rises in pitch, seems to 'crack' and needs to be cleared constantly are plain.

In the classroom pupils and students make assumptions like everyone else. The male or female teacher who is unable to control a class often cites the voice as the cause. 'My voice isn't strong, so they don't think I mean what I say.' 'They say they can't hear me at the back of the class, so they just keep talking.' Male teachers often find maintaining discipline easier than women teachers and some of this can in part be attributed to their vocal quality; the lower male pitch creates a marked acoustic contrast between their vocal output and the ambient noise in the classroom.

Male teachers who have reported problems to the authors, related to gaining and keeping the attention of the class, have, without exception, been those with a fairly 'light' vocal quality. They reported that they had to spend a lot of time forcing their voices to produce a louder, deeper sound, and often resorted to shouting; as a consequence, they developed vocal problems. Many teachers who have problems being vocally commanding resort to shouting and the effect of this is often that, far from appearing to be *in* control, they are indeed perceived as having *lost* control. Pupils often complain that a teacher 'always sounds angry and aggressive' but when questioned further this can be less the result of the content of what is said and more the result of the quality of vocal delivery.

Modulation

Modulation of the voice is an important feature of communication, of how 'the message' is put across. Teachers will often complain that their voices lack interest or modulation; they feel that the voice is contained within a very narrow range and that it does not move in response to thought or word; they feel that it should be 'modulated'. Modulation, however, is a word much used and often misunderstood. It suggests (erroneously) a technical changing and varying of the voice, with no regard for the thought that produced it. Movement of the voice through a series of cadences without reason produces a sound just as unconnected to mind and action as a dull monotonous voice. Ideally, the voice should respond to changes in thought, these thoughts being reflected by a variety of subtle vocal changes. If, however, tension or stress levels are high, it is likely that this natural delivery will be inhibited. When the individual is relaxed and at ease, the voice moves effortlessly and naturally through its entire range, the movement reinforcing the intention of the language rather than distracting from it.

Vocal colour and energy

Of course, there are aspects of emphasis to be considered such as pause, pace, pitch and stress, all of which add natural colour, energy and nuance to the voice. Their use or lack of use is usually an indicator of how open or happy the teacher is about engaging the breath and voice freely and responsively, rather than being the result of a lack of specific technique. Emphasis is always present when a speaker is clear about the message that he or she is conveying, just as energy is present when the speaker has a 'need' to be heard. You only have to listen to a group of enthusiasts debating a subject close to their hearts to understand this. Vocal colour is heard when a voice is well connected with the breath, has range and is capable of pitch change. Most individuals display their true vocal colour when they laugh. Successful classroom vocal technique can create a productive environment by combining discipline and generosity. A free, colourful and unforced sound is able to develop warmth and resonance, and to convey subtle changes of thought and emotion. A voice that clearly invites the class to enter into an exchange of ideas, while at the same time being able to define the boundaries of that exchange, is an invaluable asset to a teacher.

Pauses

Pauses are often limited, because it takes confidence to *hold your ground*, to remain silent without losing concentration, and yet crucial communication takes place in the time allowed by a pause. One piece of information should be digested before another is presented. There is often pressure to speak rapidly, to get it all said so that the class can get on with the work, when often what is being said is an absolutely essential part of the work. Pausing before important phrases, and before and after names and dates, can help listeners retain key facts. The use of the pause, rather than speaking over a noisy group, can be a valuable control mechanism.

Rhythm and energy

Rate is the speed at which an individual word or group of words is spoken. To process information effectively, it is important to speak at a reasonable rate. Pace, on the other hand, can be thought of as the overall energy and rhythm of the delivery of an entire speech, so that individual words can be spoken clearly and concisely, but the general pace can be driven forward energetically. This means that speech may have clarity, energy and precision, as well as a sense of the 'drive' of language flowing in rhythmic cadences. The most effective way of gaining confidence in the ability to use words is to practise speaking words that have been carefully selected, that trigger exciting and interesting sound patterns and images. Read aloud, for example, from the verse and prose that make up the wealth of English literature. The joy experienced when 'feeling and tasting' the vowels and consonants in the mouth is intensely rewarding. Speak passages that engender a passionate response, words that reflect personal ideas and feelings. When there is commitment behind the word the voice reflects it naturally.

Vocal spontaneity

A more difficult aspect for the teacher or lecturer to master is the ability to make old knowledge sound new. Teachers and lecturers may have taught the same course for many years, but the truly effective teacher is able to impart the information as though it was as new to him or her as it is to the class. When enthusiasm is natural, not pushed or forced, and the speaker uses breath freely, without any postural or tension problems, most of the aspects that determine an 'interesting' voice are present. Sometimes, however, a habit of sounding monotonous has developed over a number of years and, indeed, may have been with the teacher as a child or an adolescent. Habits, such as vocal monotony, can develop during a period of insecurity or vulnerability and frequently, when the phase passes, the habit may remain. For some adolescents, the idea of standing up in class and reading or speaking in front of their peers is terrifying; the jaw tightens and all vocal variety is suppressed. For others a vocal quality is assumed as part of a survival strategy, such as the adolescent 'chill', 'street cred' approach, which may involve a very limited use of range. Generally these phases are natural stages of development, but, as with posture, the muscles often hold the pattern after the phase has passed and the voice remains limited and underdeveloped.

Gesture

Gesture provides a natural reinforcement to what is being said. French and Italian speakers are perceived as using a lot of arm and hand movements to reinforce what they are saying, whereas this is less noticeable in English and German speakers. Obviously there are exceptions to every rule, but in general gesture has cultural implications and roots. This use of gesture is referred to as non-verbal communication and within this category the term 'body language' is frequently used to refer to all the means, other than speech, by which individuals communicate. These range from posture to small movements of the fingers, from eye contact to shaking hands. As with vocal variety, gesture should be the end-result of thought processes and should stem from the desire to communicate those thoughts and ideas to the listener. Imposed gesture is quickly identified as artificial. Gesture works best when the speaker is sufficiently relaxed to integrate mind, voice and body in a total gestalt. Excessive gesture distracts from, rather than adds to, the message being conveyed.

Presentation

The dynamics of the workplace are often affected for good or ill by something as simple as the clothes that an individual is wearing, the posture, voice quality and national and/or regional accent. All these aspects form part of the communication process – the way in which individuals interact with one another in a social context. These paralinguistic features will determine how an individual is judged by those with whom they come into contact and, like it or not, these value judgements, often the product of prejudice, are deeply entrenched and difficult to alter once they have been made. Within the teaching profession, value judgements made of teachers/lecturers by pupils or students will critically affect the relationship between them and influence, for better or worse, the dynamic within the classroom. The same is true, of course, among fellow professionals in whatever occupation. Students are just as likely to be victims of these judgements. Knowledge by teachers of these paralinguistic features may alleviate judgements of this kind.

Accent and dialect

Recognition should also be given to the fact that accent and dialect are often the criteria on which initial impressions are formed. Intrinsically they carry certain intonation patterns, e.g. a Welsh or Indian accent has a much more musical quality than, say, a German or Russian accent. Musicality, however, has a hidden cost; individuals with a musical accent are sometimes perceived as lacking authority. The inflection pattern, which gives the more musical sound, can at times be falsely interpreted as questioning and uncertain.

Accent and the assumptions that are made about accents are well documented (Honey, 1989) and should be challenged in the classroom, otherwise change will never occur. Nevertheless, newly qualified teachers with a specific regional accent should be aware that accent is, for some, an emotive issue. A teacher with a different accent may be positively perceived or, conversely, the difference may be the basis for ridicule, particularly from adolescent pupils or students. Younger children seem much more generous, but adolescents often take their attitudes from the 'soaps' and these do nothing to break the stereotypical assumptions of regional accent, but rather reinforce them.

The accent with which an individual speaks is usually the one spoken in the area in which they were raised and the one used by their primary carer. Today, however, so many family units move from one area to another that many children have parents with different accents or even different mother tongues. Children who move in their early years generally adopt the accent of their peer group in an effort to conform and be accepted. This transition from one accent to another happens very quickly, in some children in the period of a few weeks.

By the middle teens accent is less likely to alter; adults seldom significantly change their accents dramatically, although most individuals are 'vocal chameleons', slightly adapting their speech according to changing situations – the phenomenon of the 'telephone voice' is well recognized. Adults, however, rarely make a conscious decision to change their accent unless for very specific political or sociocultural reasons. A teacher from Leicester, whose accent is completely 'London', provides a useful example here. This teacher had taught in south-east London for many years, during which time he had consciously allowed his accent to change because he felt that it was easier for the class to relate to him. This is not a common occurrence; the richness of regional and national accents should enrich the life of the classroom and teachers should not feel a need to eradicate or seek to eradicate their accent. Nevertheless, people's accents may be devalued. A Jamaican teacher, known to the authors, provides an illustration of this. The teacher, in an attempt consciously to alter her accent, was misusing her voice. Her written comment after attending a voice care and development training course was as follows: 'felt valued as a Jamaican, I wasn't put down. Hurrah!' Whether this teacher had been 'put down' in the past because of her accent was not known, but certainly she felt that a lack of respect for her nationality was inextricably linked to her accent, and the perception other people had of it and hence of her. This small cameo illustrates the considerable significance placed on accent.

Teachers should attempt to ensure clarity and vocal spontaneity, whatever their accent, and promote tolerance in children by encouraging them to talk about the diversity of speech in the school, community and region. When children understand the reason for differences they cease to mock them.

Paralinguistic features

So what are the factors that determine first or initial impressions? Mehrabian (1972) suggested that the major component of a 'first impression' is visual, what is seen – the person's appearance, posture, body language, facial expression and eye contact. What is heard – the voice quality, the pitch of the voice, the pace and use of pause, the clarity of speech and the accent that the person has – determines the auditory component of an initial impression, whereas the words that are said are initially very low on the list. Mehrabian awarded each component a numerical score, so 55 per cent of the impression formed of others is visual, 38 per cent auditory and 7 per cent what is said. It may seem almost unbelievable that, through what appears a rather arbitrary set of criteria, decisions are made that will affect future relationships, but that in fact is what appears to happen. The validity of this form of judgement lies in the fact that most people, when asked how often they have altered their first impression of someone, will respond, 'rarely'. The first 5 minutes are indeed critical.

Rogers (1975) noted that a major barrier to interpersonal communication lies in an individual's natural tendency to judge – to approve or disapprove of – the statements of the other person. Statements do not need to be verbal; as has been said earlier, statements are made by an individual's choice of clothes, hairstyle, facial expression and body language. So how does this process work? When forming an impression of other people, an individual is influenced by a set of beliefs and values. When these values and beliefs are extreme, objective assessment becomes impossible, colour prejudice being a particularly evident and malicious example of this, as are sexual, gender and age prejudice. In forming relationships with other people individuals want to have their own ideas and beliefs reflected; there is a well-recognized tendency for individuals to 'like people like themselves'. In part, this is because 'like-minded' people can be understood and recognized and in part because the differences perceived in others can be very threatening.

Teachers, similarly, need to recognize that pupils and parents, students, staff members and school visitors make instinctive judgements at the beginning of every school year, and past pupils and students may reflect back their judgements of a particular teacher. 'You've got Mrs Bough this year. Oh goodness, she is so boring and it is really difficult to hear her.' Consequently, the received wisdom is that Mrs Bough is boring and inaudible, even if this was a value judgement made by a pupil several years before.

It is also important to recognize that the tendency to evaluate is very much heightened in those situations where feelings and emotions are deeply involved. The stronger the feelings, the more likely it is that there will be no middle ground; there will be two ideas, two feelings, two judgements, all missing each other. For teachers this situation is predictable; the pupils are anxious about moving into a new class, and the teacher is equally anxious about the new pupils. What will the class be like, will there be problems of discipline, will there be children with special needs? An incorrect assumption early on in a student–teacher relationship can determine the ongoing communication, often with critical results. After all, there are few professions where such an intimate relationship exists over such an extended period as that between teachers and their pupils.

Given the need to maximize the opportunity to communicate effectively, how can this be achieved? There are several well-recognized communication facilitators, which can be applied in any situation, as discussed below.

Facilitating communication

Positioning

How an individual is positioned in relation to another person or persons is very important; each position 'says' something. It is not always possible to choose where to sit, but the position can affect the interaction that takes place in significant and predictable ways. There is a tendency to sit opposite a competitor; this obviously has much to do with a desire and a need to be in a position to monitor the other person's movements. In teaching there is very little choice; positioning is fairly well prescribed by the number of pupils and the need to view the whiteboard, overheads, PowerPoint or audiovisual aids. In primary school this is easier; more teaching can be undertaken in a round-table setting which also encourages a more participative atmosphere, even if a noisier one. Wherever possible teachers should try to vary the placement of desks and try to encourage more participative positions.

When considering interview situations, e.g. when visiting the doctor, or someone in authority, this 'opposite position' appears to be the preferred position, although more doctors are introducing a diagonal position *vis-à-vis* the patient, which is similar to that of an 'interview' situation. Sitting or standing alongside another individual is the recognized cooperative position, but that is more rarely seen in formal situations. Needless to say, this would be most difficult for teachers to achieve in junior or secondary schools, but it could be achieved in small group tutorials or discussion groups and is certainly to be recommended.

Distance

Distance from another person or group of people would not at first sight appear to be an important aspect of communication, but it has been recognized as having a considerable effect. Studies have highlighted appropriate distances for specific communication situations. From nought to half a metre is an appropriate distance for intimate social situations, half a metre to one and a half metres for personal situations, talking to good friends or colleagues, whereas social/consultative situations require a distance of one and a half to three metres to be maintained between people. For public situations more than three and a half metres between speaker and audience is appropriate. This suggests that for most teachers and lecturers there is a positioning mix within the classroom environment. For those pupils sitting at the front of the class, they and the teacher relate at a 'personal' distance, whereas, for those further back, the relationship is one of a 'social/consultative position' distance. The result of this is a mismatch within the dynamics of the class or lecture room as far as positioning is concerned. Teachers should be aware of this and attempt to compensate for it, by perhaps addressing more comments to the back of the class, spending more time making eye contact with those at the back of the class, looking at their posture in relationship to those at the back, and indeed deliberately moving around the class so that they achieve a mix of 'personal' and 'social consultative' positioning with all pupils and/or students.

Body language

One of the interesting things to have been discovered is how individuals who are in tune mentally or who respect the other person tend to mirror each other's posture and this is a significant clue when looking at group dynamics. Those who are in tune are usually looking towards each other and reflecting back each other's posture, whereas those who are not compatible show definite signs of defensive body posture, arms crossed, leaning away and lack of eye contact. It is perhaps appropriate for teachers and lecturers to reflect on some of the current studies available on body language, which may offer strategies for them in terms of classroom management. In this way early observation of aspects of body language, which may signal disinterest, anger or depression, may be noted and contained.

Dealing with the voice of doubt

Teachers, like actors, often have to contend with niggling doubts about their own ability. This is especially difficult when a disruptive class undermines their status and confidence. Most teachers admit to thoughts such as 'I can't do this', 'I can't control this group', 'The class thinks I'm a walk over', 'This class is going so badly. It must be my fault', 'I should have prepared this better'. This 'self-speak' can be as undermining and hurtful as if it were being said by an examiner or a colleague. It is also difficult to control once it has started and must be challenged.

Many teachers speak about walking into a class feeling that they have lost the battle before they have even started. It is important to notice what such an attitude does to the body and how it subsequently affects the breath and therefore vocal use. Consider for a moment the posture of defeat and that of victory as well as the postures for well-being and depression. In defeat the shoulders round forward, the spine slumps, the head comes down and the eye levels drop. All this leads to a lost space between the hips and ribs and results in diminished breath capacity. Feeling confident and positive lengthens the spine, opens out the chest. The weight is balanced and the head is poised on the top of the spine allowing the eye levels to lift and open up peripherally. There is also considerable space between the hips and lower ribs allowing for breath to be full and low.

There are dangers of course in striding arrogantly into a situation because messages of physical aggression may be 'read' by the class, but it is important always to be aware of the language of the posture used.

How does the teacher develop a positive 'self-speak'? The first step in doing this is to acknowledge the negative self-programming that exists. Some revealing work is being done at training days given by Mary Johnson at the Educational Development Service in Warwickshire. To illustrate the point she asks a teacher to address a class while another teacher whispers negative suggestions about the performance in his or her ear. The teacher then describes how this made him or her feel. The exercise is repeated while being given affirmative ideas. The teacher is finally asked to comment on how he or she felt in both situations.

Generally teachers are able to relate to this exercise and to acknowledge that they are often undermining themselves unnecessarily. This is particularly likely when morale is low or they have been experiencing difficulties on a regular basis and so they anticipate failure before they even encounter it. It is important to look beyond the difficult situation to the teacher's desire and commitment to teach and enhance the lives of young people. By reminding themselves of their aspirations and learning to excuse the occasional badly handled situation, it becomes easier to re-discover the joys of teaching. Carrying demoralizing thinking and low self-esteem from difficult situations into new challenges can only be limiting and ultimately damaging.

Explaining

Edwards and Furlong (1978) note that: 'Whatever else he [sic] does the teacher will be talking for most of his [sic] working day.' This will occur either, as Edwards and Furlong suggest, in small groups and with individual children or, as in most secondary school classrooms or in further or higher education lecture rooms, as a public performance. Not all this time is, however, spent in simple transmission. Dunkin and Biddle (1974) estimate that the proportion of time spent on explaining by teachers varies from 10 to 30 per cent. Studies by Martin (2003) noted that teachers reported that on average they spent 60 per cent of each lesson talking. Ogunleye (2002) reported an even greater proportion of lesson time: 80 per cent spent in teacher talk across further education colleges, with student talk accounting for 17.3 per cent, and silence or non-event for 2.0 per cent of the lesson. Ogunleye's findings mirror previous findings by Wragg (1973), whose study showed teacher talk accounting for between 73 and 81 per cent of lesson time in all subjects that were observed, except for French and English.

Given these findings, it is not surprising that teachers and lecturers report vocal fatigue, but teachers additionally report that a great deal of class time is spent in re-explaining information that they have already given to pupils and students. This is not only vocally tiring and frustrating but can be unprofitable. If the quality of the explanation is poor, the time is spent ineffectually. A review of the literature suggests that good explanations are not only clearly structured, but also interesting. Interestingly, pupils' views on explaining appear to have been consistent over a period of 60 years, because Hart (1934) found that the principal reasons for liking a teacher were based on the teacher's helpfulness in terms of school work and the ability to explain lessons clearly.

Explanation: strategies and skills

Explaining can be described as a mixture of strategies and skills, which need to be mastered if explanations are going to be effective. Teachers and lecturers and indeed anyone who is in the explanation business need to remember this. Despite the 20 years that have elapsed, the strategies cited by Brown (1986) are still highly relevant. He suggests that:

- topics should be analysed into main parts
- links should be established between these parts
- the characteristics of the learner must be accounted for when adapting plans
- if there are any rules involved in the explanation they should be defined.

Brown also suggests that those giving the explanation must have certain basic skills, such as:

- clarity and fluency
- emphasis and interest
- use of examples
- organization and feedback.

Edwards and Furlong (1978) highlight the synergy of what is said, how it is said and the social relationship in which the speech is embedded. They also suggest that, even in the absence of hard evidence about what has been learned, the articulate teacher is likely to be judged effective. Comments reported by Brown (1986) over 20 years ago remain relevant. Students cited their main dissatisfaction with teachers and lecturers to be: failure to emphasize main points, failure to pitch at an appropriate level, inaudibility, incoherence and reading aloud from notes.

Clarity and fluency can be achieved through defining new terms, use of explicit language and avoiding vagueness. Emphasis and interest can be achieved by variations in gesture, use of media and materials, use of voice and pauses, and repetition, paraphrasing or verbal cueing.

Examples, when used, should be of sufficient quantity, clear, appropriate and concrete and, where applicable, positive and negative. The organization of the lecture, lesson or explanation should be in a logical and clear sequence with the use of link words and phrases. Feedback to the listener should provide opportunities for questions and there should be an assessment of what the listener has understood of the main idea. In addition the individual giving the explanation should seek to understand the attitudes and values of those to whom he or she is speaking.

Many of the above issues, which cause student dissatisfaction, are easy to remedy and could make a considerable difference to class response.

It is worth remembering that good communication skills indicate that the speaker not only respects his or her audience, but also values him- or herself.

Oral skills

For many people the thought of standing up and addressing a group rates as their greatest fear. The young people who are now pupils in schools will be facing the same fears in adult life, and it is sensible educational practice to develop their skills and confidence in the area of interpersonal communication skills. If young people are given the opportunity to gain the experience and confidence needed for easy, structured and sustained public speaking, those fears need never materialize and the adults of tomorrow will be much more effective speakers.

Too often the crowded curriculum does not allow for work of this kind, other than a token amount in the English syllabus. Traditionally, in the UK the public schools have placed great emphasis on oral skills but all children should be offered the same opportunity. Practice in oratory can be gained by reading aloud from public speeches by the great orators as they teach about effective structures. Debating societies, drama groups and involvement in reading and addressing assemblies all offer an opportunity to gain these skills. Business and industrial courses are currently teaching simple formulae for effective speech. Although they are a wonderful starting point, they are easily identified and the devices of manipulation are often obvious. Atkinson's (1984) study of oratory and politics makes fascinating reading for anyone wanting to understand and improve the structure of formal speeches. The information that it offers is undoubtedly useful for teachers and lecturers.

Above all teachers should be supported in working on their own voices. The teacher who is aware of the role that the voice plays in communication is clearly advantaged. Kathy, an experienced teacher and trainer explains her relationship to her voice and her craft:

> *How I sound, whether I am shrieking and pushing the voice or sounding dull and monotonous, will affect the students at an unconscious level. I need to be able to read all the clues: If I am breathy it may be that I am too reliant on what others are thinking. If I am not finishing my words this has something to do with a lack of trust in what I am saying.*

> *If my pitch is restricted I am not playful. Pitch is released by a sense of joy and diminished by a lack of it. Teachers in the primary school often tend to have more playfulness in their voices than the teachers in the secondary schools. If I try to control through a rigid, inflexible pitch it eliminates a sense of fun and a sense of freedom. When my body is relaxed enough to allow a free and varied use of pitch, it also has open resonating spaces so my voice has resonance.*

Control is seen as such a highly desirable thing in the classroom, and so sometimes I control in the wrong way and the consonants are held on to and the vowels are lost. This leads to the control being there in the voice but the feeling and empathy is not. Discipline is necessary but in our 'culture of control' we often forget to share the control with the children. If I share the control with them they are in control of their learning.

If we can read these things in ourselves, we can read our students better. Teaching is hard, and I have learned that you need to have access to all of your self and if your voice is locked it means that all of you is not accessible. The teacher has to be so many things to the class and the current role is often conveyed by the voice, both by non-verbal language and by the tonal quality and music of the voice.

Checking focus intention and sharing in the classroom

The following checklist serves as a reminder of the vocal aspects of communication discussed in this chapter. When we mean what we say and use language generously to evoke an interest and response in the listener, the voice is generally the easy result of a connected physical and mental impulse.

- Poor posture cuts us off from the people with whom we wish to communicate. It also places tension and strain on the vocal mechanism, and results in slumped ribs, which in turn result in insufficient breath pressure.
- If the desire to communicate is genuine and important to the speaker, the speech is usually clear and defined.
- To develop clarity a regard for the power and value of language is essential.
- The desire to share information, but not impose it, results in a free voice and clear speech. If the speaker is clear and enthusiastic about a subject the energy will transfer into the words, phrasing will be meaningful and the tone will invite listening.
- If we cut off the breath we cut off our connection with our emotions and so we are less able to communicate fully with others.
- Held breath means held ideas and so the vocal process is not integrated with mind and body.
- If the voice is forced the pitch and tone of the voice suffer. The jaw becomes clamped and the resonance is lost. The assumption made by others is that the speaker is angry or irritated and they often react negatively.
- If the voice displays tension the class will react to it; the use of a free, open vocal quality can diffuse situations and bring a positive energy to the room.

7 Words in the classroom

Words words words

In the classroom, most of the communication between teacher and student is word based. Anecdotal reports from teachers suggest that many feel that their vocal problems arise from the profound difficulty that they have with finding and using words effectively. Voices tend to work best when what is being said is important to the speaker and subsequently stimulating to the listener. Teachers are often conscious that their difficulties began as a result of a lack of focus on oral skills in their own education and feel that they would like to offer a richer language environment to their students. It would seem appropriate therefore to use this chapter to offer suggestions for raising the verbal profile of the classroom

The teacher and lecturer use words, either spoken or written, in almost every activity that that undertake. Language and its delivery underpin the way that knowledge is imparted. The modern approach to the process of education is a two-way exchange of ideas between teacher and student and therefore depends on the ability of both to participate effectively Society, however, is moving increasingly towards a use of technology that does not encourage interactive verbal skills. Although the ability of children to use technology is essential, it is imperative that the balance is redressed by the equivalent development of interesting and useful speech and language skills.

The effects of technology

Schools, colleges and universities are becoming more dependent on technology as a method of teaching. It is seen as a way of releasing teacher from contact time and often provides an effective method of instruction for subjects such as (ironically) languages. The growth of e-learning is increasingly used to provide students with a learning medium that may be conducted entirely on their own – interaction is limited to that of the computer screen. Lecturers use PowerPoint presentations supported by handouts.

Today's children are used to interacting with computer technology and obtain both entertainment and information from screens. Although the educational value of television cannot be under-estimated, the result of young schoolchildren spending time as passive *viewers* rather than active *doers* has, however, reduced reading time and has led to an erosion of the broad range of expression available to children. Many children entering school are unable to use language to communicate; they do not have the experience of conversation at home, and nursery and primary teachers are expressing concern about communication skills in the early years. Children are prevented from accessing the curriculum because they are unable to communicate. Considerable amounts of Government funding have been and are being awarded to *Sure Start* schemes in areas of social deprivation in order to give specialized communication skills training to help to prepare children for the educational environment.

Older children, similarly, may display limited language skills; teachers increasingly report that their students are using language mechanically and automatically, that they are using words without thought. For this reason, many teachers express a keen interest in returning to the teaching of oral skills, skills that provide society with the opportunity to enjoy words and foster a delight in the speaking of well-ordered and expressive language, skills that have been 'sidelined' by the crowded curriculum.

It is important to be clear that the move is not to reinstate old-fashioned, class-based 'elocution' classes. These can be divisive and may restrict language rather than free it. What many teachers want is to encourage a move towards ensuring that children of all cultural backgrounds are not disenfranchised because they are not given the language skills that allow them to express their needs clearly and achieve their goals. There are several organizations that have worked tirelessly over a number of years to promote such work. The English Speaking Board, founded by Christabel Burniston, has done much to stimulate an interest in spoken language. It offers examinations in oral communication for schools, colleges, commerce and industry. Public speaking festivals and competitions organized by the English Speaking Union have also contributed to the development of the 'oracy' skills of the young people who are fortunate enough to attend a school that participates. There are also many local festivals that promote the speaking of verse, prose and reading as a performance skill and even broadcasting. In many schools teachers of English take responsibility for productions and festivals within the school, but with the loss of the specialist the time-consuming task means extra unpaid work for the generous volunteer.

Spoken English in the curriculum

Undoubtedly the more discursive approach to spoken language allows teacher–student relationships to become proficient in informal conversational practice, but it is critical to recognize the power of the formal structures that underpin oratory. The National Curriculum in Britain now has an element of spoken English in the General Certificate of Secondary Education syllabi, but this is not enormously challenging or demanding for many verbally able students. The inclusion of English literature as well as English language as a compulsory subject has been welcomed by all. However, it is not only the pupils who need consideration and help with the delivery of language but also the teachers, who in many instances feel that they too would benefit from help both with their own skills and with devising ways of stimulating discussion and verbal analysis.

Ideas from outside

Apart from the excellent published material available there are currently many opportunities for staff and students to receive an injection of new ideas and stimuli from outside organizations. Some theatre companies run workshops on the plays that they produce and offer follow-up packs with suggestions for both written and oral exercises. In the UK, the Royal Shakespeare Company has an Education Department, which not only gives workshops for students on the current season and sets up residencies in schools, but also runs an annual Shakespeare School, which is designed to meet the needs of teachers teaching Shakespeare at GCSE and A level. This brings together the three overlapping worlds of theatre practice, contemporary Shakespeare scholarship and educational practice.

Making words physical

Young people are often discouraged when faced with language, which to them seems alienating. By entering into language physically and by speaking words out loud and putting their analytical skills aside for a time, a fuller, more meaningful understanding is achieved. Helpful exercises in this approach can be found in *The Actor and the Text* by Cicely Berry (1993), who began working with teachers and young people over 30 years ago. Through her need to find ways of making the language of the classics accessible to the young, she has made a seminal contribution to the teaching of language in schools and formulated an approach that involves the whole class actively entering into the language physically and vocally.

The experience of speaking the texts is all too often overlooked in the classroom situation, where the good readers are generally the only ones who get the opportunity. The Globe Theatre in London has an Education Department doing text-related work, as does the Royal National Theatre and many regional and fringe theatres. Theatres in other countries run similar outreach projects. Although the work that they offer may not specifically focus on speech and language, the work is all practical and drama based, and will encourage debate in addition to helping the teacher with less experience of drama explore unconventional approaches to text and language teaching.

Finding help

For teachers who feel intimidated by having to read verse, prose and dramatic texts aloud, there are classes held through Adult Education Courses that may be useful, such as a drama group or a public speaking class. Toastmasters and other similar societies offer opportunities to develop skills in formal speaking. Popular at present are groups that offer the opportunity to explore story-telling, oral history and reminiscence, all skills useful to the teacher, and skills that can be used to enrich the oral tradition within the class. Some people prefer individual classes and in the UK, the Society of Teachers of Speech and Drama provides a list of recognized teachers while similar societies exist in other countries. There are often workshop advertisements in theatrical and professional journals, which are available at larger libraries.

In-service training days

When a group of teachers from one school identifies the need for help in a particular area, it is usual to approach the school administration and request sponsorship from the Staff Development Fund or arrange an in-service training day. Maths and science teachers may have finished with English lessons after GCSE and certainly some of them feel that their facility with words would be supported by workshops in the use of language. For the infant and primary teacher, illuminating learning through speech as the 'story-teller' is enormously useful in developing a 'way with words'. There are those teachers who have come to the profession because of a natural instinctive skill in communication and even performance. In many institutions, the skills of the advanced level and technical teacher are closer to those of the university lecturer than to those of the classroom teacher, where teaching may involve delivering long tracts of memorized material. In these cases the style of teaching is closer to public speaking. The art of the public speaker is needed in these instances and is explored in Chapter 10. Developing an interest in debating can enhance this skill, and there are teachers and lecturers who have learned to deliver speeches effectively through the experience of having to run a debating society, or by entering groups of students into public speaking competitions. Many who take on this responsibility complain that they are not being given the training that they need for what is an essential part of their job. Where only a few teachers from a school require a specific workshop it is sometimes possible to approach the local teachers' centre which could provide training.

Special language needs

In the infant school the acquisition of language is rapid and the child explores words and masters syntax through books, stories and play, which become a significant way of making sense of the world. The classroom is an ideal setting for the development of the pupil's ability to use language. It is the place where teachers will recognize early indications of problems in language development or in the acquisition of speech sounds. The child's parents or primary carer, because of either a lack of experience or simply a lack of appreciation of the problem, may have overlooked these signs. Familiarity often makes it difficult to 'isolate' a problem; it is part of the child's repertoire of speech sounds and is, as such, unremarkable.

An increasing number of children now attend playgroups and nursery schools and here language and speech are fairly closely monitored. Playgroup and nursery school leaders are increasingly aware of the problems that can occur. Fortunately there is ever more awareness of the work of the speech and language therapist and the intervention that is available, yet there are still a number of children who are overlooked. There are instances where children have specific phonological problems that parents will not accept as needing treatment, or that they perceive as being rather appealing, such as /th/ rather than /s/ being used or /w/ substituted for /r/. The problem for the primary school teacher is that, if the child is unable to perceive the difference between one sound and another in speech, it is even more difficult for him or her to perceive the difference between one sound and the other when reading, and of course an appreciation of phonics is an essential pre-reading skill.

In the same way, subtle difficulties with language, on either the expressive or receptive side, can be overlooked and only come to light at school entry when there is more need for the child to use language to express more abstract thoughts and ideas. Issues of receptive language difficulty such as semantic relationships, word classes or oral directions, or of expressive language, such as recalling sentences, formulating sentences or sentence assembly, can have been overlooked and only become apparent when having to use language in a more precise form.

Children learn some of their early speech skills from repeating what they hear, and from nursery rhymes and songs, which, because of their rhythm, rhyme, harmony and disharmony of different combinations of vowels and consonants, are easily committed to memory and these verses remain with them for the rest of their lives. It is unfortunate, however, that it is these specific skills that are reportedly being lost as a result of a decline in communication skills within the family circle, caused by a variety of sociological factors. These include changing social and familial patterns, e.g. reduced contact with the extended family, increased isolation, reliance on television and computer use, lack of family mealtimes. Changing working practices often reduce the time for parent/carer/child interaction. Concern about child safety imposes more rigid supervised social interaction, reducing opportunities for spontaneous play, such as playing in the street.

Although the overarching policy of inclusion in schools is commendable, the increased number of children with special language needs within the classroom, such as autism and hearing disorders, imposes an increasing burden on teachers and support staff, and may indeed reduce the teacher's ability to find time to focus on children with less severe speech and language disorders. Although volunteers often provide assistance in the early stages of reading practice, teachers should alert the volunteers to the early warning signals of speech and/or language delay. It is often these 'helpers' who have the most one-to-one contact with the child. The Royal College of Speech and Language Therapists offers advice in recognizing speech and language problems and may be contacted to locate the local clinic or specialist centre.

Language opportunities in the secondary school

Exploration of ways of opening up debates with adolescents is an area of considerable interest to teachers. Adolescence is a time when alternative views are normal and it is important that schools recognize this and allow ideas to be expressed through debate and discussion. Speaking the words of others is often the first step to being able to find words for oneself. English literature offers such an enormous variety of wonderfully honed and precisely constructed examples of the expression of every conceivable emotion. When offered to young people for exploration and consideration, such verse or prose often releases the words within individuals and allows their own thoughts to be manifested in language. The more interactive and vocal the English class becomes, the better. Teaching students to appreciate and 'own' literature can be wholly successful only when they experience the speaking of it. Many adolescents have needs that they are not able to express or deal with adequately, such as feelings of rage and grief, huge enthusiasms and devotion to particular groups or individuals. If teachers can help students to express their needs and help them to find the words with which to make some sense of their lives, then true education takes place.

Although some of the opportunities for the use of verse and prose with adolescents have been mentioned, all age groups from the playgroup upward can use these devices. All too often, verse is used only by the English teachers and in drama, but the opportunity to use poetry in history and social studies, and in fact in almost every class in the school, is often sadly neglected.

Choral speaking

Choral verse was a popular way of teaching children verse up until the 1970s. It has lost popularity because it was seen as being taught for all the wrong reasons. At one stage it was used as a way of imposing 'received pronunciation' on children who had regional accents, and therefore discarded. There are, however, many positive reasons for encouraging classes to speak together, the most important of all being simply that it offers many children who are not exposed to verse the opportunity to come in contact with it and to experience the physical joy of speaking verse. There is always a danger that the teacher will feel the need to make the children sound 'correct' rather than allowing them to feel the energy and the sound of the language, the sheer enjoyment of telling the story, and communicating the material to the audience. The act of speaking together develops empathy between members of the choir and a sense of team spirit similar to that developed through sport. The demands made by the exercise go far beyond the simple act of memorizing words.

The speaking of well-selected verse demands the development of a feeling for rhythm that informs the child's own speech and writing and his or her appreciation of rhythm in verse and prose. It also offers the valuable experience of speaking language rather than analysing it. This adds a physical and organic dimension to work with words at any stage. A group can also explore verse by taking a line each around the classroom, responding to the vocal energy of the words and of each other, and developing a communal voice. Working towards sharing of work with other classes and parents can be an enriching experience for all, but it is sometimes a mistake to concentrate on the performance of group verse rather than simply speaking it for its own sake. The process should always be more important than the product.

Speaking words that are carefully chosen to be part of a well-shaped and honed structure, and part of an overall intention to be communicated, take the words beyond the page and 'into the mouth', so that the pupils know what it feels like to speak them and not just to read them. The speaking of powerful words leads to the empowerment of individuals and the understanding that the words that are presented on the page have enormous power and influence to change people, situations and ultimately lives. The person who can express him- or herself in words feels in command not only of language, but also of his or her life. The frustration that often leads to violence can, instead of turning in on itself, be channelled through language both to become a positive creative force and to lead to a better understanding of self and others. Berry (1992) says, 'For when you cannot speak, what is there left but violence?' There are many psychologists, welfare workers and teachers who would agree with this, but in the need to equip young people with writing skills the spoken word often gets neglected. The need to develop the oral skills of society is obvious, but who takes on the burden of the additional teaching?

The loss of the specialist

A common complaint among teachers is that, with the loss of the specialist positions of the speech and drama and music teacher, many teachers find themselves undertaking a role for which they have had limited preparation, teaching subjects in which they did not originally specialize. Teachers feel justifiably under-confident in teaching a class and a discipline for which they have limited training or qualifications. Some teachers feel a pressure to accept additional duties and are fearful of admitting that they are not able to teach either speech-based work or singing. This is a situation illustrated by the following example of a teacher who, because she was the only member of staff in her village school who played the piano, found herself teaching singing. She commented: 'The worst aspect of teaching singing was that I was so embarrassed at having to demonstrate. Eventually, after becoming extremely anxious about it and on occasions feeling that my throat completely closed up, I went to a wonderful singing teacher at my own expense and gained some confidence. I now enjoy it.' The demands are increasing, and the school should offer the proper training by means of in-service courses for anyone in this position.

Singing

Although most singing teachers do a wonderful job in the musical life of the school, some singing teachers of the past have much to answer for where children have been adversely affected and in some cases scarred by thoughtless and often ignorant remarks. Teachers will recall (often, and probably not coincidentally, those experiencing vocal problems) humiliating remarks made to them by class or singing teachers about their supposed 'inability' to sing. It appeared that these remarks were followed by suggestions that they should not sing, but rather 'mouth' the words. Such remarks are never child centred but are usually concerned with the teacher's, or the head teacher's, desire to produce a 'polished' performance for an adult audience. Suggestions to a child who finds maths difficult simply to refrain from completing the lesson would be seen as irresponsible, so why should it be acceptable to prevent some children from singing, when what they need to improve their pitching is more practice, not less. With enough practice and positive encouragement, the child who pitches normally in speech can be given the confidence to pitch accurately in song. Singing should be a natural, joyous and fundamental part of every child's education and as with choral verse the process should be more important than the product.

A recent study at the Institute of Education (Ward, 2003) showed that parents who criticize or laugh at their children's attempts to sing or play an instrument risk turning the children off music for life. The study, mirroring the teacher's anecdotal comments above, suggested that an adult's dislike of music can usually be traced back to a 'disapproving experience' of making music as a child, either at home or at school. The researchers at the Institute of Education said that even a throwaway remark from a parent or teacher can 'foster a sense of childhood or adolescent musical inadequacy and shame that can persist into old age'.

The teaching of singing to young children, who in many cases have hearing that is not yet sufficiently sophisticated to pitch accurately, should also involve teaching them to listen through a series of auditory training exercises. These lessons in listening will have a positive effect in many other areas of school life. Singing can also provide excellent practice in speech sounds because definition is required and produced when the children are committed to the act of singing.

The singing lesson, as with the choral speaking lesson, offers a wonderful opportunity to establish the essence of easy, free, spontaneous voice use. Children can be encouraged to align themselves well and stand with the weight on both feet and with a long spine. They can be taught to 'breathe down' rather than to 'take a big breath', to release the shoulders, relax the jaw and keep the head balanced on the top of the spine.

The opportunity to establish these fundamental principles should not be lost. Being part of a group that is involved in the creation of communal sound is a wonderful experience, whatever the age of the pupil or student. Much has been written about the act of singing and the loss of this essentially primal social activity from our culture is to be deeply regretted. In selecting material for song as for verse, it is important to reflect not only the majority school population but also to embrace minority cultures within the school. Music and verse can greatly enhance empathy with other cultures and other countries. The singing of traditional songs allows children to enter into the narrative tradition and to develop an interest in story-telling that is often lacking in the modern family unit. It can provide a useful way of extending work on other languages and may naturally engage with different subject areas, such as history and geography.

Children who stammer sometimes find great freedom in song, as the process of singing, particularly in a group, allows them to enjoy the experience of communication without the stress that many of them find in speaking on their own. Many adults who stammer report that they rarely, if ever, stammer when singing, in the same way that many find talking to animals and small children a relatively stammer-free experience. Within the classroom teachers are often uncertain how to approach the child with a stammer in order not to marginalize them from speaking situations, but at the same time not to force them to speak in situations that they find difficult. It is important to try to establish, with the speech and language therapist, the best approach for each child.

Many children with special needs will enjoy the rhythm and participative nature of song. There is a significant body of knowledge now available through the work of music therapists, which will offer a way into language through music for children with special needs.

The value of singing goes beyond the technical aspects of breath, pitch, communication and precision of sounds, because, as with all language, its delivery is a gestalt, involving body, breath, mind, intention, rhythm, musicality and interpretation. It develops not only musicality, but also the interpersonal and ensemble skills of group timing, anticipation and cooperation. For many children the act of group speaking or singing allows them a great deal of freedom to explore their own creative powers and imagination.

8 Vocal health

A perennial topic raised during teacher workshop discussions is how teachers can most effectively limit vocal strain within their working environment and how best they can maintain vocal health, given the demands of the classroom. This chapter explores some of the personal strategies that teachers can adopt to preserve their voice and prevent potential vocal difficulties.

Early warning signals

What are some of the early warning signs that teachers should be aware of? A worrying concern is the lack of attention that early warning signs of vocal abuse and misuse receive, despite efforts to highlight voice care within education through the efforts of organizations such as the Voice Care Network. Notable developments have been the endorsement of the Voice Care Network's publication *More Care for Your Voice*, by the Health and Safety Commission's Schools Education Advisory Committee (SEAC) (2003). The General Teaching Council for Scotland has produced a document about voice in the teaching profession, the only teaching council in the UK to have done so and the Department for Education and Skills (DfES) in their Healthy Schools Healthy Teachers (2001) website recommends that teachers and trainee teachers should be referred to specialist help from a speech and language therapist and/or an ear, nose and throat (ENT) consultant should they experience vocal problems.

Although these initiatives are very much welcomed, vocal health information and education are still not given a high enough priority within teaching. Martin (2003) found that 92 per cent of those within her study reported that fellow staff members did not see voice care as important. One reason for this may be the number of teachers in every staffroom experiencing similar voice problems. The unspoken message is, therefore, 'this is a problem we all expect to have at some time or another; it will probably improve so don't worry about it'. In view of persistent funding difficulties, teachers are very reluctant to take time off work, with what could be perceived as a fairly minor ailment. This is a familiar situation in many schools and underlines the commitment of the majority of teachers, who endeavour to 'keep going', irrespective of the state of their voice. As a result, the serious long-term implications of a voice problem may not be seen as demanding particular attention and may most regrettably be disregarded.

Early indications of vocal misuse and abuse

For many teachers the first indication that they are abusing or misusing their voice comes not as a specific voice production problem, but rather as a feeling of tightness and tension in the neck. Teachers report that they are aware of their throat feeling rather stiff; some describe this as a feeling of generalized 'soreness', whereas for others the feeling at times is one of considerable pain. Teachers and lecturers have indicated, anecdotally, that there is tendency to ignore such symptoms, ascribing them to tension or stress. They may, however, be early indications of undue effort accompanying vocalization. When voicing is effortful a major contributory factor can be undue tension related to habitual posture and muscle state.

Postural implications

In addition to the fundamental postural issues discussed in Chapter 5, it is important to monitor specific classroom postures, which can become habitual and lead to chronic physical and vocal problems. An obvious problem arises from the height of the desks in the infant school, which requires the teacher to spend sustained periods of time leaning over while speaking to children or marking their work. Many people who have spent significant amounts of time in study appear to be unaware of poor head and neck alignment, which may lead ultimately to kyphosis or what is often referred to colloquially as a 'Dowager's hump', frequently to be seen within the older population. This results from a loss of alignment between head and neck and, as a result, the curvature of the spine at the level of the cervical cartilages becomes pronounced. This, in turn, leads to an alteration in the head–neck–spine relationship and changes to the position of the larynx within the pharynx. Constriction of the larynx may occur and changes in the configuration of the pharynx and the vocal tract may result in a rather 'squeezed' pharyngeal sound. If possible, the teacher should crouch beside pupils, or draw up a chair alongside the child when explaining or helping with work.

It is important for the teacher or lecturer to try to monitor his or her posture in different activities throughout the day, such as when working at a desk or computer or when giving instructions to the class. Ideally weight should be kept well distributed across both feet, with knee joints flexible and unlocked. Standing with arms crossed should be avoided, because breathing is restricted and the body tends to slump forward. The spine should be long, the pelvis should be level, with space between the hips and lower ribs, and the shoulders 'low', with the neck free and the head well balanced on the top of the spine.

Apart from the postural implications in terms of stress and tension sites, rounded posture has an effect on communicative intent; it portrays someone who appears to be lacking in authority. In non-verbal communication terms a speaker with an easy upright posture is often perceived as much more authoritative. In addition, good posture provides support for the voice quite effortlessly, reducing the potential for vocal abuse and misuse.

Very small changes in posture may make a significant difference, e.g. half-spectacles, often prescribed for those individuals who need them only for reading, tend to encourage people to look up and over to see what is happening within the classroom, and this 'up and over' posture alters the neck, head and shoulder configuration. When working on the upper body, teachers often report little awareness of a habitually high shoulder position, apparent only after attempting to work on relaxing this area. For many teachers a high shoulder position never alters, whether driving, reading, walking or sitting. By raising the shoulders, the space within the pharynx is limited and the larynx is constricted, so voice is produced much less easily.

Taking time during the working day to think about shoulder position is worthwhile. The following questions provide a useful benchmark:

- Is it possible to lower the shoulders?
- Are the shoulders relaxed?
- How much space is there between the base of the skull and the shoulders?

In Chapter 11 a range of exercises is suggested, several of which will help with postural change. For individuals who drive to work through busy traffic, the tension experienced en route can be established for the rest of the working day. Using the time to counteract the build-up of tension by lifting and releasing the neck and shoulders when an opportunity arises, e.g. at traffic lights, or in the ever-increasing traffic tailbacks, is recommended. Good driving posture should include support to the lower spine, not impose tension on the shoulder girdle, and maintain a released head and neck position.

Sitting

The 'sitting' bones or ischium bones serve the same function as the feet and it is therefore important to remember to use these bones to provide adequate support and balance when sitting. Although classroom practice encourages teachers and lecturers to embrace movement rather than maintaining a fixed position, it is important, if sitting for long periods of time, to pay attention to the seating provided. Seating in schools is not always comfortable and uncomfortable seating not only imposes back strain but also exerts pressure on the abdomen: when slumping forward breathing is restricted, when slumping backwards pressure is put on the lower spine. Chairs should offer adequate support for the back and should be at a good level when working at a desk. As a guide to height, Macdonald (1994) suggests that the chair height should allow an individual to reach the surface of the desk comfortably. In addition when both hands are flat on the surface the arms should be bent at a right angle. When writing at a desk, table or keyboard, Macdonald suggests that one of the first requirements is to use a sloped surface, which creates far less strain on the wrists. A piece of board, or a tray with a support behind it, can be used to make a sloped surface. When using a computer, the keyboard should be angled through the use of a support behind or customized keyboards may be purchased. Reported incidents of, for example, repetitive strain injury (RSI) or postural and eyestrain through extended computer use have encouraged many institutions and authorities to develop health and safety documentation to cover these issues, which are to be welcomed.

Many teachers and lecturers prefer to stand during lessons and indeed some schools and colleges do not encourage staff to sit when taking lessons. Standing for long periods is, however, very tiring and staff may often lean against a desk during teaching periods. This posture is not to be recommended, because there is a tendency when leaning against a desk to do so with one buttock on the desk and one leg supporting the weight, thus throwing the body out of alignment and preventing easy supported breathing for speech.

Teachers have frequently been caricatured as individuals clad in academic gowns and weighed down by piles of books. Undoubtedly many teachers and lecturers do have to carry far too much material, particularly if they do not have an assigned work-station or classroom, and have to move around the school or college campus with teaching materials. Bulky papers or assessments are often marked at home and need to be carried out of school or college.

Within the classroom, large amounts of material needs to be kept 'available' for projects, which involves the teacher moving boxes of stationery, equipment and project material from place to place. As with carrying heavy weights, the potential for damaging the lower back is high. In the same way clearing out deep cupboards and high shelves can be difficult for teachers. The best way to carry heavy weights is close to the body, cradled against the chest or, if a substantial amount of material has to be carried, it should, if possible, be divided into two piles, with the weight distributed equally, otherwise undue strain will be imposed on the spine and lower back (Figure 8.1).

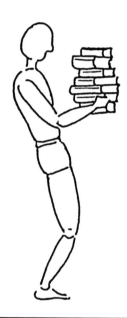

Figure 8.1 Incorrect carrying position

Teachers with chronic pain or tension should invest in themselves, in terms of treatment. When the problem is chronic rather than acute, a series of massage sessions by a properly qualified practitioner, or work with an Alexander, Feldenkrais or Pilates teacher, can do much to improve the situation, and prevent vocal problems resulting from poor posture. When muscles are damaged in some way (and problems in the neck, upper back or shoulder area can easily occur), an instinctive protective response is initiated and this, as noted in Chapter 4, can result in discrete changes within the skeletal and muscular framework that will affect voice.

Monitoring of body posture can distinguish between what is normal and what has become habitual and, once highlighted, postural problems are not difficult to deal with. For some people, achieving the 'new' posture is initially easy but difficult to maintain; achieving change does take time and awareness. Considerable effort has to be expended to make the 'new' seem comfortable and, until established, far from seeming better, posture may indeed seem rather worse. Consultation with an alignment professional from one of many physical strategies available may be the most effective way of changing poor habitual posture.

Self-monitoring

Tension and effortful voicing may be the result of difficulty in appropriate self-monitoring of the voice. Without training it is very difficult to assess voice volume levels accurately. The instinctive response when trying to make oneself heard is to increase volume and indeed at times shout 'over' noise, as noted by Comins (1995). Teachers report that when a class is making a lot of noise they try to take control by increasing the effort that they put into producing the sound and endeavour to 'push out' the voice. For untrained voice users this is not only hugely tiring, but also counterproductive. Martin (2003) noted that primary teachers reported using their voice at high volume for the majority of their lesson time, thus imposing considerable strain on the vocal mechanism.

Individuals can be trained to shout easily, without straining the vocal folds, but, for most teachers and lecturers, being trained to shout is not necessary; instead, what is important is to acquire alternative skills that vocally or non-vocally 'cut through' the noise. This may be through the use of a vocal pitch that is higher or lower than the ambient noise or, to limit the strain on the voice, the use of an instrument such as a cymbal or tambourine may help.

Much of the shouting that occurs in school or college is very damaging to the voice and indeed very tiring. It is also quite difficult for pupils, many of whom find constant shouting distracting and at times distressing. In an ideal situation shouting should not be necessary, but even the most resourceful teacher resorts to this very human reaction on occasions. For the teacher concerned, the extreme vocal effort may manifest as pain and tension in the neck, and occasionally in the jaw and tongue. The vocabulary of pain or discomfort is very personal, and although it is difficult to 'translate' these feelings, novice or reluctant singers may experience a similar effect in an effortful attempt to maintain a note. A feeling of tightness in the neck and particularly under the jaw can result, caused by tension in the large tongue muscles, which form a 'strap' under the chin. The point of insertion of these muscles is the hyoid bone, which, as already noted, has an intimate relationship with the positioning of the larynx within the throat. Changes in this positioning will in turn affect the movement of the vocal folds.

For many teachers this feeling of tension is a daily occurrence; for some this tension although quite exhausting does not create permanent vocal problems, but, for many, the legacy of such daily effortful voicing is either vocal damage or a reduction in the range and robustness of the voice.

Loss of range

Many teachers report that they no longer have the singing range that they used to have; nor can they make themselves heard over the normal classroom noise. Indeed some teachers report that they cannot make themselves heard at the back of the class (Martin, 2003). Although these teachers may have never experienced partial or complete voice loss, they have experienced a significant diminution of their vocal range and vocal effectiveness. One of the difficulties of this type of chronic vocal abuse and misuse lies in the fact that, for many teachers and lecturers, the problem has been slow and insidious. It is only when teachers are asked to think back to their vocal function at the beginning of their career and compare it with their current ability that they appreciate how much their range has diminished. Had the change in voice quality and reduction in range been either more sudden, or more complete, then more attention might have been given to the problem, allowing the teacher to retain much more vocal flexibility.

Personal strategies

There is much that can be done to reduce vocal abuse and misuse through the use of simple strategies. The following strategies are effective in reducing vocal damage.

Liquid intake

Every teacher should ensure that they drink more than the national average! It is important to drink at least 1 litre of water, bottled or tap, sparkling or still, per day, in addition to that contained in the normal intake of liquid through drinks such as tea and coffee. Tea and coffee have a diuretic effect and as such can be dehydrating, so it is important to 'top up' with water in order to maintain the moisture level within the body at an optimum level. Indeed some specialists would suggest avoiding tea and coffee completely and substituting herbal teas. The maxim 'pee pale' is a good rule to follow; urine that is pale in colour indicates a good level of hydration in the body. (For those on medication it is useful to remember that vitamin B makes urine darker in colour.) Although drinking cannot directly lubricate the vocal folds, an increased fluid intake will increase the general body fluid level and prevent dehydration.

It is particularly important to keep the fluid level topped up when the vocal folds are in any way vulnerable, e.g. in women of menopausal age, where as has been seen the vocal folds are subject to tissue change, as well as in those individuals who are heavy smokers or drinkers. While recognizing that there are health and safety issues regarding water in the classroom and the imposition in certain schools of a rule preventing teachers drinking while teaching, it is most important for teachers to endeavour to keep water at hand, if at all possible. One solution is to introduce a humidifier into the classroom to limit atmospheric dryness, or to encourage the installation of a water dispenser in the school.

Teachers and lecturers who are working on the Information and Design Technology syllabus should try to remember to wear a mask if working on materials likely to create dust, with lathes or saws. Small dust particles are very irritating to the vulnerable larynx, as are paints or varnishes. Teachers who are taking swimming classes in heavily chlorinated swimming pools should be vigilant in case of possible adverse reactions.

Steaming

Steaming is a very effective way of introducing moisture into the vocal tract in an effort to minimize some of the dryness experienced as a result of colds, vocal fatigue and stress. The tried and tested method of inhaling steam by leaning over a bowl of hot water (it is not necessary to add herbal extracts to the water) is very successful or, alternatively, have a long shower remembering to inhale the steam, preferably through both the nose and the mouth.

A useful and perhaps more practical alternative is a nebulizer or steam machine, which allows moisture to bathe the vocal folds and reduces dryness in the respiratory tract. Nebulizers are currently available from high street chemists at a reasonably moderate price. It is important to remember that these machines must be cleaned out meticulously after use, because fungal infections can occur if the machines are not properly and hygienically maintained. The use of distilled water is recommended and oils or herbal preparations should not be added to the machines. It has been suggested that maximum benefit is incurred by using it three times a day for five minutes at a time. Steaming immediately before giving a long presentation or performance is an excellent anti-abuse preventive measure. Many actors and singers use steam regularly to keep the vocal folds lubricated while the effects of hydration on the vocal folds have been the subject of several published studies (Verdolini-Marston et al., 1994). Increased hydration levels will affect the speed and ease with which the folds move, which has an important effect on voice quality. It is also important to remember that in the process of vocalization heat is generated by the action of the vocal folds, which, in addition to the drying properties of overheated classrooms, increases dryness in the vocal tract.

Smoking

It is not the purpose of this book to proselytise on behalf of the anti-smoking lobby; the negative effects of smoking are well known, but perhaps less well known are the negative effects of smoking on the voice. Smoke irritates the respiratory tract and specifically affects the vulnerable vocal folds. Upper respiratory tract irritation and sinus and asthma problems can all be exacerbated by contact with smoky environments. In terms of vocal health it is important not to smoke, but, if it is impossible to give up, a reduction in the number of cigarettes smoked is recommended. It is encouraging to note that most schools and educational establishments are smoke free; others offer a separate smoking area.

Diet

During the past decade, increasing importance has been paid to the effect of gastro-oesophageal reflux on the general condition of the vocal folds. This is where gastric acid from the stomach is regurgitated, spills into the larynx and bathes the laryngeal mucosa, resulting in irritation to or inflammation of the mucosal linings (Jones et al., 1990). Any change to the structure of the vocal folds alters their vibratory characteristics, leading to change in vocal quality. In instances of gastro-oesophageal reflux, the structural change in vocal quality is perceived acoustically as hoarseness. This perception of hoarseness may encourage the individual to increase vocal effort in order to overcome the hoarseness and this in turn may compound the vocal damage.

Digestive problems may occur without an individual being aware of them, so undiagnosed and untreated gastro-oesophageal reflux may be present and not recognized unless specifically assessed as part of a full vocal assessment. In instances where gastric reflux has been identified, it is particularly important for individuals to avoid eating late at night, in order to maximize the time spent in a vertical position, during the digestive process. The distance between the upper end of the digestive tract and the larynx is approximately 20 cm, so, in a prone position, there is more likelihood for gastric acid to seep into the larynx and cause inflammation and ulceration. One remedy is either to sleep on raised pillows or to raise the height of the bed. Spicy or highly seasoned food, fats, coffee, chocolate, smoking, alcohol and 'gassy' drinks can all aggravate the condition. It is important to be aware of food or liquid that is likely to cause adverse reactions and to avoid it if possible.

The effect of acid reflux on the vocal folds with associated voice quality changes may also occur as a result of frequent vomiting. Teachers, lecturers, parents and carers should be aware that changes in voice quality might indicate a bulimic condition in young susceptible adolescents both male and female.

Various types of food may contribute to thickened saliva and dryness of the mouth. Spicy food, for example, may result in thirst and a dry mouth, whereas foods with high carbohydrate content or thick milky sauces, often lead to sticky thick saliva. A dry mouth and thick secretions will encourage regular throat clearing, leading to irritation and potential damage to the vocal folds.

Throat clearing

Throat clearing and coughing are often the presenting symptoms of vocal abuse. Many individuals are quite unaware of how often they cough or clear their throat, but the sensation of having a 'frog in the throat' or a 'tickle' is one that is frequently cited by those with voice problems. Unfortunately the process of 'clearing' the throat has quite the opposite effect because in coughing the vocal folds are brought together with considerable force. In turn, the vocal folds, in an effort to reduce the ensuing friction, become bathed in mucus, which the individual then feels the need to get rid of by clearing the throat, and so the problem continues. One way to limit this vicious circle is to keep a supply of water available and try to sip some water rather than clear the throat; the action of sipping the water appears to limit the need to clear the throat and gradually the problem becomes less acute. If it is not possible to sip water try instead to swallow, rather than cough.

Hard attack

Hard attack, where the vocal folds come together forcefully at the onset of a word beginning with a vowel, is the result of a lack of coordination between the initiation of voice and the initiation of breath. A common characteristic of the speech of stressed individuals, it manifests as a hard initial explosion of sound especially evident in phrases where words begin with vowels such as, 'All right Class 8, I said quiet!' The explosion of sound that can be heard is caused by a lack of synchronization of the muscles of breathing and the muscles of speech, resulting in the vocal folds coming together with great force, which may, over a period of time, damage them. If this is an established habit it can be remedied by allowing a little breath through the vocal folds before speaking, e.g. adding an /h/ before the word 'all right', so that it becomes 'h-all right', takes the stress off the initial sound. Practice in saying lists of words beginning with vowels in this way encourages a more gentle onset of the note and helps the muscles of breath and voice 'remember' the appropriate posture and effort level required and, once this action has become familiar, it should be enough simply to 'think' /h/ before vowels to reduce hard attack. Habitual vocal patterns tend to be strongly entrenched and therefore, in order to achieve vocal change, it is important to persevere with exercises for some time. Chapter 11 gives details of this and other exercises.

Cold remedies

Individuals anxious to avoid the need to take time off work frequently use over-the-counter cold remedies, which are designed to eliminate excess moisture and 'dry up' a cold. These cold remedies contain a high level of caffeine, aspirin and often antihistamine. They are certainly effective but, for professional voice users such as teachers and lecturers, the drying effect on the vocal tract, allied to the vocal demands of the role, is difficult to reconcile. There is always a conflict between taking time off work with what appears to be a rather trivial illness and 'soldiering on', but it is important to remember the damage that can result from 'forcing' the voice even for short periods.

If the voice is to be used strenuously and at a high volume over a period of time, it is advisable to use paracetamol and not aspirin as a remedy for colds and flu. The blood-thinning properties of aspirin can, in some circumstances, contribute to haemorrhaging of the vocal folds. Sucking throat lozenges and pastilles should be kept to a minimum, because they often contain strong dosages of decongestants that can affect the vocal tract. It may be worth noting that mentholated sweets that can be bought over the counter have a very limited effect on the mucosal lining of the nose and although they may seem to 'clear' the nasal passages, they would appear to be more of a panacea than a cure.

There are of course occasions when it is impossible to take time off work and so short-term remedial pharmaceutical measures can provide short-term symptom relief, but long-term use is not advised. It cannot be stated too forcibly that any vocal change persisting for longer than 2–3 weeks after a cold should be reported to a doctor.

Allergies

Given the increase in over-the-counter medication it is not uncommon for individuals to self-diagnose and, without seeing a general practitioner, to self-treat for a variety of conditions including hay fever or common nasal allergies. For many these remedies work well but for others even a mild nasal decongestant may have a negative impact on the nasal mucosa. Frequent use of sprays for allergies without advice from a pharmacist or general practitioner as to the pharmaceutical content is not recommended. Professional voice users should ensure that medication is appropriate and does not have any unwanted side effects that may contribute to vocal attrition.

Clothing

Classrooms, school and college premises are extremely difficult to heat to a constant temperature. In the early morning the classroom is usually quite cool, with the temperature warming to a muggy heat by the time the last bell goes. As a result, teachers and lecturers often find that they are cold when they come into work and remain cold for some time after starting work, especially in older premises that are not well insulated. When cold, blood vessels contract to maintain as much body heat as possible and cold muscles do not work as efficiently as they do when warm. In an effort to conserve heat the tendency is to limit movement and indeed individuals may often be seen 'hugging' themselves to retain body heat. A useful tactic is to wear layers of clothing, so that as the room heats up a layer can be divested and a steady degree of warmth throughout the day can be maintained. Clothing that is too tight, particularly across the chest and back, can impede breathing by restricting the degree of rib expansion and in the same way wide belts that are pulled too tight will constrict the diaphragm, particularly when individuals are seated, thereby limiting effective respiration.

Physical fitness

The link between voice and physicality has already been explored in Chapter 5, but it is important to remember that keeping flexible and mobile is very important, not only for long-term health, but also in an effort to underpin and maintain effective respiration, reduce areas of tension and encourage vocal flexibility. Counteracting some of the effects of ageing on the skeletal framework is also to be recommended, because effective and efficient use of the voice is possible into old age, providing that supple rib movement is maintained in order to aid respiration and conserve good spine, pelvis, head and neck alignment.

Yoga classes are a particularly useful way in which to focus on relaxation, breathing and general muscular flexibility. Low-impact aerobics, as well as encouraging physical fitness, will also contribute to increased respiratory function. Keeping fit has the additional benefit of releasing endorphins, which influence mood swings and generally are thought to contribute to a feeling of well-being, as well as discharging tension. For many people who find exercise classes tedious, a creative alternative form of exercise could be a dance class. If formal classes are not of interest, regular walking will improve breathing, strengthen muscles and bone, and improve stamina. Swimming will serve the same function and is particularly good for the muscles involved in respiration; swimming has the added benefit of being totally impact free, which is of relevance to the older individual and particularly relevant to those who may have osteoarthritic or rheumatic joint conditions.

Warming up

As with any form of intense physical activity, it is important for teachers and lecturers to warm up vocally before beginning a day's teaching, a vocal equivalent to a marathon. Athletes warming up before a race are rarely seen running on the spot; most perform an initial series of stretching exercises that gently encourage muscle movement and only then do they start to jog, or run slowly, but never do they run at full stretch as part of their warm-up routine. Teachers and lecturers, however, once they begin work, rarely do anything but the equivalent of 'running at full speed' vocally. To spend time gently vocally stretching and making contact with the breath is important. Mersbergen et al. (1999) suggest that vocal warm-up leads to an increase in blood flow to the muscles and an increase in nutrient deposition to the muscles used. As a result exercised muscles have increased activation potential and possibly improved fine motor control; in effect they work better. The vocal warm-up exercises included in Chapter 11 are very useful preventive measures against vocal abuse and misuse, and are to be recommended. Warming up can be brief and subtle and can be carried out almost anywhere. Humming a tune gently and sliding up and down the range on the sound /n/ or /m/ is a low-impact vocal exercise that can be carried out almost anywhere, from sitting in the car to walking down a corridor.

A strategy for warming up is to involve the class, if the pupils are of an appropriate age, by doing exercises that both relax and energize everyone. This can be as simple as the game of 'Simon says', in which the instruction is carried out only if prefixed by the phrase 'Simon says', e.g. 'Simon says raise your arm', 'Simon says jump up high', 'Simon says stand on tip toe' and so on, to a modified series of exercises that allow the children to move around the room, even if only in designated areas. An all-over stretch is very beneficial and can be incorporated into classroom activities without disrupting the teaching routine. The stretch allows the children to alter their positions, which not only prevents them from getting stiff but at the same time releases tension, which might result in the children fidgeting and losing concentration. The stretch in fact re-focuses the children's attention and does not, as might be thought, prove distracting. Remember that postural habits can become fixed during pre-adolescence, so any input reaps the double benefit of helping the class and the teacher. There was a time when physical education in schools actively promoted postural awareness, and it is regrettable that this is no longer the case. Any individual effort on the part of the teacher should be seen as a bonus for pupils.

Voice care

The following information serves as a reminder of some of the strategies discussed:

- Do not try to talk above loud background noise at social or sports events or above machinery noise
- Avoid smoking
- Avoid chemical irritants or dusty conditions
- Try to keep alcoholic drinks to a minimum
- Do not respond by shouting when upset or anxious
- Avoid excessive use of the telephone
- Be aware that spicy foods and dairy products may affect your voice
- The voice is closely linked with emotion – tension or depression will be reflected in the voice

- The voice needs moisture – keep up your liquid intake but avoid excess alcohol, which dehydrates
- Pale-coloured urine indicates a good level of hydration
- Warm up the voice gently before prolonged speaking
- Avoid dry atmospheres – use a humidifier or water spray to moisten the air in centrally heated classrooms, offices or homes; if you have conventional radiators a wet towel draped over the radiator effectively humidifies the air
- If your voice is hoarse or you are losing your voice, do not whisper or try to continue talking; rest your voice
- Be aware of voice quality
- Monitor any change in your voice carefully and see a doctor if there is a persistent change in quality
- If you are having continuing vocal problems, ask your doctor to refer you to an ENT specialist or otolaryngologist.

9 Effective classroom strategies

Repertoire of strategies

Chapter 1 identified the heavy vocal loading that teachers experience in primary, secondary and tertiary education; Chapter 8 identified ways in which personal strategies could be adopted to reduce vocal strain effectively. This chapter offers ideas and suggestions that can be used so that teachers and lecturers may formulate a repertoire of classroom strategies to overcome or at least alleviate some of the factors inherent in classroom practice that may contribute to vocal abuse and misuse. It is recommended that teachers and lecturers collaborate with colleagues in building up a library of suggestions suitable for their particular work place, which can be kept in the staff room and displayed prominently so that the staff focus on the issue of health and safety.

Ventilation

A number of common causes of vocal abuse and misuse have their origins in environmental conditions that are endemic to school life. Although it may not always be possible to change conditions, it may be possible to mitigate them by, for example, following certain rules of vocal hygiene and voice care. Avoidance of laryngeal irritants is an important factor in vocal hygiene. The laryngeal mucosa is extremely sensitive, so it is important, where possible, to avoid smoky, dusty atmospheres. Teachers and lecturers frequently work in buildings where ventilation is a problem, often because the windows are hermetically sealed and cannot be opened, even partially. During winter, when the central heating is turned on, classrooms can become too hot, and a very dry atmosphere will affect the respiratory tract and the larynx. Air conditioning can have the same effect, so it is very important to be aware of the possible effects on the voice and to take steps to lessen the problems.

Common classroom infections

Inadequate ventilation contributes to a hot dry atmosphere, which is damaging to the voice and in addition contributes to the spread of infection so that coughs and colds abound. It may be necessary to have a well-documented procedure for minimizing the spread of coughs and colds. In the primary education sector, teachers could request that children not be sent to school if they have very heavy colds but, if this is not realistic, try to separate the infected from the non-infected to limit cross-infection. A plentiful supply of tissues should be available in the classroom, which children should be encouraged to use.

Attempting to limit infection is important because repeated colds can be particularly debilitating and many teachers report that their voice first showed signs of deterioration after a bad cold. The recommended vocal management in the case of a cold or respiratory infection is to try to talk as little as possible, to look after the voice by drinking plenty of water, and steaming and resting it. Instead of continuing to talk to the class throughout the day, it is important for teachers to indicate that they have a cold and need to talk less. The need to find effective ways of dealing with the limitations of a cold can positively develop teaching styles. The strategies outlined below are particularly effective for use with younger children and are designed to help to encourage the class to develop 'good looking' and 'good listening' skills.

Attention skills

Small children often have poorly developed listening and attention skills; they may also have problems of auditory immaturity and these are areas that teachers often focus on in infant and junior school teaching. Teachers should try to encourage children to look and listen for signals, which are not necessarily vocal. It is useful to begin each term and half-term with a refresher session where the teacher recaps on the procedures involved in listening and looking. Highlight the importance of the child's active involvement in this process and the need for him or her to remember to look and listen to the teacher throughout the day without prompting. Asking for the class's attention is a frequent daily occurrence; rather than saying or shouting this instruction, teachers may like to try using an alternative non-vocal approach, e.g. a large cardboard hand on a stick with

'Stop' written on it can be raised to indicate that the class must be quiet and await instructions. Cardboard traffic lights on a stick with the stoplight painted a vivid red can be used as well. Encouraging children to keep a watching eye on the teacher is good for working on visual attention and developing 'good looking' skills.

Cymbals and drums can be used to signal silence on the part of the class; when the sound is heard the class must stop talking and be quiet. Another useful device is a 'round robin' message, which follows a well-designated pathway. The teacher gives her request to Child A, who is nearby; Child A passes on the message to Child B, and so on around the class. Ask the last child for the message and compare this with the response of the first child. The class are always anxious to let the last child know if a mistake has been made, but the message can range from 'Be quiet' to 'Put your books away and stand in line'. By making a game of it when the teacher is 'in good voice', it is established as an accepted procedure that can be used most effectively when necessary. By highlighting the importance of listening, improved listening skills can be encouraged and voice conserved. For teachers with severe voice problems using a hand or throat mike or indeed fashioning a megaphone from cardboard can be a useful aid.

Hearing

Teachers will all be familiar with the problem of hearing impairment in pupils. This may range from a degree of hearing loss that requires hearing aids, to intermittent deafness caused by recurrent middle-ear infection, commonly known as 'glue ear'. For some primary school children this can be a source of continual absence from school and indeed, because of the fluctuating nature of middle-ear infection, a child may be able to hear clearly one day and not the next. Speech and language disorders are also common in the primary school population. These can range from relatively minor problems to much more severe problems of language acquisition and use, to problems with sound production, which is where work on auditory attention is undoubtedly useful, because it encourages the child to focus on the auditory, rather than the visual, channel.

Teachers also should have their hearing tested periodically, because, with increasing age, from 50 onwards, hearing acuity becomes less. Any diminution in hearing may be almost imperceptible from one year to the next, but the cumulative effect over many years can make it difficult for teachers to hear pupils, or to distinguish what is being said if there are a number of children talking at one time. Teachers who have to listen above the noise of machinery such as drills or saws, or indeed home economics teachers who have to listen above the noise of electric beaters or sewing machines, will find this particularly difficult if they have any degree of hearing loss. Some hearing loss will also have the effect of making it difficult to self-monitor the loudness level of conversational speech.

Arranging the classroom

Positioning the class with care is very important. Remember that lip-reading is an important additional factor in aiding understanding. Lip-reading is an instinctive process when listening to speech, which is why there is often a need to ask for repetition of specific information on the telephone, and why confusion arises with certain phonemes; it is not unusual, for example, to hear, 's for sun, not f for Freddy'. If pupils can be seated so that they can see the teacher's face when he or she is giving instructions, it will greatly aid understanding and reduce the level of loudness required by the teacher. It is important for male teachers to remember that moustaches and beards do make lip-reading more difficult so they will need to compensate by articulating clearly. When working in acoustically difficult spaces, children should be grouped, which will provide a damping effect so lessening the need for excessive volume on the part of the teacher.

Positive teaching styles

Arrangement of the class or lecture room should allow for the free movement of both pupils and staff. It should allow the teacher or lecturer to stand beside or behind each pupil or student when teaching and make verbal, visual or physical contact with each child. Recent work within the classroom has shown that a teacher can modify 'bad' behaviour by walking up to the child, putting a hand firmly on the child's shoulder, exerting gentle pressure and saying nothing. 'Nagging' is deeply wearying for teachers, may lead to accusations of bullying and seldom changes the student's behaviour; rather it may simply inflame a difficult situation and create a rather fruitless and negative atmosphere within the classroom. Teachers recognize their own tendency to 'nag' but report that it has often been difficult to find alternative effective responses, so this is seen as an encouraging development. Members of the teaching profession will be very aware of the guidelines regarding physical contact with pupils and students, so this is an approach that needs to be used with care and confidence, in order to avoid any potential misunderstanding of intent. It is obviously inadvisable to use any form of pressure that could be interpreted as pushing, jostling or threatening.

In attempting to maintain order in class, teachers report that their greatest resource is their ability to observe and assess the mood of the class and to remain vigilant without becoming reactive to the class's manipulation. Most teachers find that objective observation allows teachers to change the class's behaviour without losing respect and cooperation. When teachers were questioned, most reported that they found talking, deliberate hindering, idleness and pupils being out of their seats the most annoying aspects of class behaviour, specifically because it is these behaviours that considerably reduce teaching time. Students and pupils are quick to observe vulnerability and disruptive elements among the student population will inevitably try to capitalize on this.

It is obviously important to maximize positive response, reinforce good behaviour and minimize negative responses. When the negative response is used sparingly, its effectiveness is considerable; when used constantly the effectiveness is minimized. Teachers and lecturers admitted, when questioned, that their reinforcement of positive attitudes to academic standards far outweighed their positive attitudes to social behaviour. Positive reinforcement of social behaviour is important otherwise lack of effort is associated with positive reinforcement in a negative way. It is often common to comment on lack of effort rather than praise pupils who continue to do what they are told without causing any trouble. Positive reinforcement should be used with honesty so that children see it as genuine and well deserved; they quickly see through 'phoney' praise and this therefore invalidates real effort.

Teachers and lecturers will be very aware of the importance of approval and disapproval to pupils and students but in the often-frenetic atmosphere of the classroom it is sometimes difficult not to 'reserve' approval for really major effort, and focus more on instances of wrong-doing.

Negotiation skills

A major cause of stress develops as a result of poor negotiation within the classroom setting or the staffroom. A great deal of tension can be defused by the application of effective negotiation strategies. A major cause of adolescent rebellion and staff discontent comes about through the frustration that results when individuals find themselves in 'no win' situations. The old-style authoritarian approach places people in the position of feeling that, if one person wins, the other loses. Negotiations that work to find 'win/win' agreements (where both sides feel that they have won) rather than 'win/lose' situations leave everyone happy and productive and cooperative as a result.

Young people who, quite rightly, are being taught to 'know their rights' often have difficulty understanding that other people also have the same rights, problems and needs. On the one hand, they are told to 'be assertive' and 'learn to say no', but, on the other, they are accused of being 'self-centred' and 'stubborn'. Assertiveness, when it does not take the needs of others into consideration, becomes a form of bullying. It takes maturity to be able to find the workable solution to problems that seem irresolvable. Most adolescents have a highly developed sense of justice and can therefore easily relate to the fairness of the 'win/win' negotiation.

To bring about such an agreement, it is necessary to break through the deadlock that is the result of individuals being unwilling to accept the other person's point of view. Concessions often need to be made and these should be made on both sides. When one party is expected to concede too much without due recognition and discussion of their needs, the result is a breakdown in communication, feelings of resentment and a withdrawal of goodwill. Such situations benefit neither party and serve only to increase general stress levels.

Negotiation skills can be learned from books or better still by the organization of a staff development or in-service workshop. The information gleaned from such training can be passed on to students by the application of strategies to the classroom situation and formally within the oral element of the English class. Many schools have Personal and Social Skills classes and these skills could be usefully shared in such an arena. Schools with specific problems such as bullying and racism can apply the principles of 'win/win' negotiation in order to bring about understanding and reconciliation. The teacher who is able to apply the principles of fair negotiation to a difficult discipline problem could find that, not only has the specific problem been solved, but also the change in tactics alters the atmosphere of the classroom for the better, and indeed influences the group culture within the school. While a confrontational situation exists there will be no winners and the teacher's voice will suffer.

For many teachers, the most difficult time to maintain discipline is as the children come in and go out of the classroom. Keeping the children outside the door for a little longer and giving instructions at that time is worthwhile, e.g. 'go in quietly, sit at your desk and get out your books' is more effective than trying to give instructions as children come into the classroom, when the level of noise is much higher and teachers have to fight against this to make themselves heard.

Teachers questioned for a television programme were very aware of the 'good day/bad day syndrome' and were able to offer opinions as to why these occur. There was agreement that negative responses tended to occur when teachers were ill-prepared for the class, unsure of their material, or under external and personal stress. Teachers recognized that their mood was often dictated by a wide variety of situations, but it was particularly important to allow sufficient recovery time from a previous situation. If, for example, there was a lack of recovery time from the effect of family tensions, a difficult journey to school, an unpleasant incident in the previous lesson or an early morning staffroom rush, this could impinge on the entire school day. It is important to remember to try to break this type of pattern or at least to be aware of situations that can precipitate it and, if possible, to make changes to allow more recovery time. Lecturers and teachers may recognize that it is important to delegate activities, to admit to needing help and to try to use all possible means of reducing areas of tension within one's working environment, but finding a way of achieving this is very difficult.

Acoustics

Teaching rooms, halls and other spaces such as lecture theatres, drama studios and laboratories vary tremendously in size and design. Teachers may find themselves spending the whole day in one space, a situation common in the primary school, or working in a variety of spaces, each of which creates its own specific acoustic. Teachers and lecturers in secondary and tertiary sector find the latter situation to be the norm.

The structure of buildings and the materials used inside them determine their ultimate acoustic quality. Acoustic science is extremely complicated but there are, however, simple guidelines that can assist the teacher or lecturer in the use and, if necessary, the alteration or adaptation of a space.

It is important to observe the size and shape of the room, the texture of the flooring, the height and shape of the ceilings, and what the ceiling surface consists of. Note the number and position of windows and other glass surfaces, the material used for window and door frames, the presence of wooden or steel beams, the furnishings (steel or wooden cupboards), chairs and the substances used to cover walls, such as the texture of paint, notice boards, drapes, posters, curtains, pull blinds or Venetian blinds.

In general, and obviously all manner of combinations exist and operate differently in different spaces, low ceilings, carpeted floors, covered walls and soft furnishings tend to 'dampen and deaden' sound and absorb the voice, making it more necessary actively to voice consonants and pitch the voice appropriately, sometimes slightly higher. By contrast, hard surfaces, such as varnished timber or wooden tiles, steel-framed windows and doors, large expanses of glass and bare walls tend to produce a bright, sharp and occasionally echoing sound. This acoustic may require a change in pitch; a lower pitch may help, and a slower pace, because the reverberation of the sound can interfere with the next sound, making speech indistinct.

Both these extremes, the 'dead' one and the 'bright' one, tend to be tiring and difficult to work in. Teachers complain that working in a difficult acoustic adds to the feeling of hard work. They report that their voices are swallowed up by the 'dead' sound and, in response, they push the voice, consequently ending up feeling vocally tired. From the student's point of view the consonants, which carry the meaning of words, can be lost and therefore intelligibility is decreased. In such circumstances particular attention paid to the consonants will make a difference. A small benefit for the teacher or lecturer is that classes can sound slightly quieter, because the acoustic absorbs ambient classroom noise as well.

In the brighter acoustic, the reverberation may distract teachers and lecturers, and this proves very tiring for both teacher and class. A bright sound is exacerbated by a large area, as any teacher who has attempted to have a band or orchestra rehearsal, or a choral verse rehearsal, in a large echoing space knows. The reverberation can make timing extremely difficult and any space used for such purposes should be adapted by the installation of absorbent tiles and/or lowered ceilings.

Modification of a difficult space is not always easy and where cost is going to be incurred professional advice should be sought. There are, however, certain inexpensive adaptations that can be made.

If the room is 'dead':

- Remove any materials such as coats (hanging on pegs) and unnecessary notice boards
- Consider removing the carpet, provided of course that the floor surface is reasonable
- Remove any books that are lining the walls of the room if possible.

If the room is 'over-bright':

- Introduce screens made of an absorbent material
- Cover the floor with a soft surface such as cork tiles, carpets or a soft vinyl
- Lower or pad the ceiling with absorbent material
- Introduce more absorbent material such as drapes and bookshelves
- Cover walls in mounted artwork.

When working in large spaces teachers and lecturers may encounter problems unrelated to design, but related to the natural loss of sound over distance. As noted in Chapter 1, sound waves decrease in strength as they move away from the point at which they are initiated. To prevent the loss of the power of sound, it is important to decrease the size of the space by sectioning off the teaching area, using reflecting screens. The typical gym hall found in sixth form colleges and secondary schools is often used for a number of activities. When touring theatre companies perform in leisure centres, school halls and other non-theatre venues, they generally transport a staging area that has a false ceiling. This ensures that the acoustic they experience each night is not too badly affected by the ever-changing environment. False ceilings do not produce an ideal acoustic but are nevertheless very effective. They are obviously not cheap and prices vary according to size. An acoustic adviser or sound engineer should always be consulted before any construction of this type is considered; they will be able to give an independent opinion as to the most effective modification. Parents, and school governors, are a wonderful resource; there may be an expert associated with the school.

When working in any space with a difficult acoustic, it is always advisable to consider the students' ability to support what they hear with information gleaned from what they see. As has already been noted, there is an element of lip-reading in all the understanding extracted from speech, provided of course that the speaker is seen. In the theatre it is well known that a production that is inadequately lit is more difficult to hear, as is one in which the staging prevents the audience from viewing the actors from the front, but is presented with a profile or a back view as in, for example, 'theatre in-the-round'. Sections of the audience therefore have to listen without the benefit of seeing the actor's face. Problems of this type can be caused by poor sightlines in an auditorium and similar situations can occur in teaching spaces, when, for example, class or lecture rooms are wide and not sufficiently deep. Concentration, understanding and hearing are always limited by too oblique a view or poor visibility. Traditionally, communication takes place face to face but the communicative potential of the whole body should not be disregarded.

Visual feedback plays a significant role in listening to speech over a background of noise; in these circumstances the lips, tongue and facial muscles, and gesture should be used to communicate meaning, rather than using excessive volume. When talking over too high levels of background sound, vocal strain can quickly occur because it is difficult for an individual to monitor his or her own vocal effort and volume levels. The techniques used by actors to overcome this problem involve an omnidirectional awareness of the entire audience and a mental communication with them. Technically, concentrating on final consonants and consonants in general is usually beneficial.

Finding help

When a vocal problem occurs it is necessary to investigate the cause fully. As well as curing any symptoms of vocal stress, it is important to make adjustments to lesson preparations and their delivery so as to eradicate the underlying reasons for the stress. Stress, as noted in Chapter 3, has a very negative effect on the voice, yet stress as a result of policy and practice at different levels within the teaching environment is pervasive within education. Martin (2003) noted that policy and practice at different levels within the teaching environment contributed to pervasive identified levels of stress within education: stress at the macro level – resulting from Government policy; at the meso level – resulting from school/college policy; and at the micro level – resulting from teacher/lecturer practice and classroom factors.

Many education authorities have expert advisers whose job it is to offer advice and support. At Warwickshire Education Support, Mary Johnson works with teachers experiencing difficulty. Here she offers an example of a typical case study:

> *When I am asked to give support to teachers in difficulty, I usually observe and assess the teacher in the classroom and then consult with subject specialist advisers, so that we can offer the teacher practical strategies in order to overcome the problems. An example of this is a young teacher I was asked to help whose subject was science. She had been criticized for her lack of vocal strength as well as the content and delivery of the lessons. She was not losing her voice but her vocal approach was not effective.*

> *The year 8 class was lively and the school was difficult. There were several things that immediately put her at a disadvantage. First, the tables were fixed and the layout of the classroom created a poor teacher–student relationship. The space was large and the 15 students were spread about the laboratory behind large tables. The separation that occurred meant that there was no cohesion to the event; consequently the group did not take the lesson seriously. Their reaction was not conscious, but they perceived this from the relationship and began talking. The teacher talked over them and they talked over her. Her breathing changed, probably as her 'self-talk' became more and more negative. As she lost her breath control the voice became shriller. She tried not to shout, but as her frustration grew she began to shriek at the class. As the lesson progressed she lost confidence, began shouting over the class and the natural musical quality of the voice flattened out and became strained and inflexible. She needed help to change the relationship with the class and the dynamic within the classroom.*

> *She was given help with the physical arrangement of the classroom, and the content and the structure of the lessons. It was important that she changed the balance between her excessive speaking and the lack of verbal contribution from the pupils. It was important that she devised a way to get the pupils to feed back information so that she needed to speak less. She also needed to prepare individual learning plans for each child, including work on their own and in pairs. She had to acknowledge the battle as a battle that she must win, and in order to do so she had to refuse to speak over the class.*

She was given support in creating imaginative and inclusive ways of developing a more positive and productive relationship with the class. This helped her working life, but I had observed that there were personal issues that needed to be addressed as well. Her home life was stressed; she was coping with two young children and a demanding husband. This meant that she did not spend any time on herself, attending to her own needs or enrichment. I had noticed that her natural and unstressed vocal quality was musical and discovered that she had been a singer. I encouraged her to find time to start singing again as a way of investing in herself, developing her confidence and reclaiming the musicality of her voice. I did not feel it was appropriate in this instance to suggest she saw a counsellor.

At Warwickshire Education Support, we are introducing courses on Emotional Intelligence. These courses are concerned with 'learning about me', which is an area that we need to develop. We need to make learning about 'self' and 'people skills' central to education and educators. Then we open the way to learning about performance as an element of dynamic and effective teaching and begin to notice the role of the voice and of expressiveness in the classroom.

Help is available through education authorities, teachers' unions and a number of other interested agencies. Head teachers and colleagues are usually very willing to help and have often experienced similar problems. It is sometimes easier to speak to an outside agency and a list of agencies appears in the appendix.

10 Beyond the teaching role

This chapter explores some of the additional duties that teachers and lecturers may have to take on as part of their professional role. Each of these duties imposes vocal demands additional to those encountered in the classroom.

The chapter offers practical guidance and is intended to provide pragmatic user-friendly solutions and suggestions, some of which come into the 'quick-fix' category; others will require longer-term attention to achieve lasting change.

The teacher as orator

Within this role the teacher may be expected to address the school assembly, lead the prayers, give a moral speech, convey the daily information to the assembled school, be prepared to address a governors' meeting, welcome the audience to a play or music evening, and possibly address a gathering of parents on matters pertaining to the children's education, such as changes in education policy, choosing secondary education and fund-raising.

To give a good speech it is most important to take time for preparation. Hoping that when the time comes it will be possible to 'come up with something' will not work. The terror of having to speak is halved the moment preparation begins. With confidence the voice will behave normally, although obviously a little tension or 'stage fright' is absolutely natural, and even useful, because it provides the adrenaline rush, the edge that may be described as 'sharpening the wits'. Teachers and lecturers address groups all day, every day; it is what they are good at; nevertheless this can sometimes be forgotten in the anxiety of the more formal arena of 'giving a speech'.

The use of a clearly defined note structure, along the lines of a composition structure, with a beginning, middle and an end, is advisable. As a useful 'rough' measure, the middle of the talk should carry 60 per cent of the message, and the beginning and end 20 per cent each. It is a great help to both speaker and listener if the main points can be clearly signalled and a framework developed that contains the focus of the speech. Obviously the skills of oratory are specialized ones and much has been written that will help those who wish to extend their competence in this area. At the most simplistic level, the recommendation to 'tell them what you're going to tell them, tell them, then tell them what you've told them' is valuable.

Often the teacher's duty is to welcome a speaker, or to thank one, so it is advisable to undertake some research beforehand. The speaker's background and achievements should be included in the introduction. If the teacher's duty is to thank them, notes should be made during the speech and the salient and most memorable points reiterated at the end. Even an informal occasion such as an address by a guest speaker can produce considerable tension in the individual who has to officiate. The voice can feel as if it has 'seized up' in these moments of pressure. The question is what can be done in terms of self-help? The answer is, quite a lot.

The most important point is that the speech should have been practised a number of times, preferably to a real 'audience', be this a partner, a friend or a colleague if possible. It is important for it to be spoken aloud, not for it to be practised silently or gone over in the individual's head. If there is no opportunity to practise with an audience a tape-recorder may be used for playback purposes, but without an audience it will be difficult for the individual to rehearse the experience of communicating with an audience rather than listening to him- or herself.

When rehearsing, make sure that the body is well aligned, with the weight distributed across both feet. Shifting the weight, from one foot to another, gives the audience the immediate impression that the speaker is ill at ease. Standing firmly, but without tension, not only looks better, but also allows the individual to feel more in control.

If there is a microphone available, it is important to ensure that it has been tested and it works before it is used. Audiences find it disconcerting when a speaker taps a microphone and asks whether they can be heard, and the process will often undermine the speaker's confidence. A trial run is very important, allowing the speaker to find the best position in relation to the microphone and experimenting to achieve the most acceptable volume. Nothing is worse for an audience than to be blasted with sound, or for the speaker to find that most of the speech has been inaudible.

As a general rule it is not advisable for speakers to take a lot of papers up on the podium with them. There is a danger that notes may be lost among other papers or, worse still, that they may be dropped. Most importantly, a speech should not be learnt 'parrot fashion'; it is important to have notes as guidance so that if, through anxiety, part of the 'script' is forgotten, the speaker can glance at their notes which will prompt him or her to move to the next point. When speaking it is important to speak directly *to* the audience not *at* them; eye contact should be made with members of the audience and time should be allowed for pauses, so that significant points can be digested. Above all, the voice should maintain the speaker's natural inflection and intonation pattern. It is important to remember that the odd slip is not the end of the world; the audience is generally on the side of the speaker and wants him or her to succeed.

The teacher as sports coach

Within this role the teacher may be expected to work out of doors in all weathers, shout to encourage the team, issue instructions and caution unruly behaviour. It could also include teaching swimming in a large indoor pool with a very poor acoustic, being a cricket umpire during the hay fever season, teaching physical education, gym, dance or aerobics, and having to speak while demonstrating.

A problem produced by the need to vocalize while exercising is that less breath support can be given to the voice when lying down than when standing up, and much of the aerobics and gym teachers' work is demonstration led and floor work predominates. The number of aerobic exercise teachers who experience voice problems is high and far outweighs that of dance teachers.

Sports duties are likely to present the most vocal challenges. The cold of the rugby, soccer or netball pitch is a problem because, as has already been noted, when people are cold, they tend to raise their shoulders and tighten the neck and jaw, pull back their head and fold their arms across their body. This physical position is not conducive to easy efficient voice production. The open space is another problem. There are no hard vibrating surfaces for sound to bounce off, so the voice fades as it travels over the distance, and as a result the teacher shouts. Shouting in itself is not a problem; it is after all a natural activity – children shout joyously in the playground – but unfortunately the 'art of shouting' is something many adults in the western world have lost. In many cultures shouting is still commonplace – it is not seen as aggressive – but in British and some other cultures it is perceived as being related to anger or frustration. Chapter 12 looks at healthy shouting, a technique well worth learning for anyone who needs to project loudly over distances out of doors.

Some helpful suggestions when using the voice on the field are:

- If possible use a megaphone. This may be quickly made with a piece of cardboard. If this is not possible, the hand should be cupped around the mouth and the speaker should try to 'call' rather than shout.

- Remember that this is not a war, it is a sport. Keeping a healthy voice is much more likely if a sense of humour is retained. In laughter the voice is wonderfully free; the joyous 'Yes!' produced by a supporter after their team suddenly makes a brilliant move after playing abysmally is very different from the exasperated 'Come on!' before the successful event.
- Wear warm clothing, scarves and gloves to keep warm; warm up if necessary by exercising. Take a team near to a wall or keep them close in order to use a more conversational voice level when coaching.
- Do not battle against the wind; if the wind is blowing it is unlikely that the speaker will be easily audible. Children are more likely to understand a speaker who is clearly mouthing the words. The use of a control, such as a whistle, or flags, or a signalling system that is understood by the children is recommended in order to preserve vocal health in difficult sporting situations.

The teacher who has to teach swimming has the least enviable job! The acoustics in indoor pools are invariably poor, because of the abundance of hard surfaces and high ceilings. Often they are echo chambers and the space becomes incredibly noisy, particularly if the classes take place while public or shared sessions are occurring.

In such a situation it is difficult to offer helpful advice, because many teachers report not only that is it a most difficult task but also that it causes enormous vocal tiredness. Some teachers have reported that, with improved general voice production techniques and the use of non-verbal ways of controlling the group, it has been possible to cope better. As with field sports, the use of a control to minimize voice use is important; whistles can be high-pitched enough to pierce the noisy acoustic, although problems occur if other teachers use them in shared sessions. Using a flag to get children to swim to the side can be effective, but often a sound signal will be needed as well. A variety of signals should be taught to the children, e.g. one long blast means 'stop', two short blasts means 'come to the side'.

Small children and non-swimmers should be taught only in a quiet environment and in small groups. All children should be clearly instructed on what to do when they have completed a length, so that they look to the teacher for advice before proceeding. It is pointless to expect children to hear anything when their heads are in the water.

Teachers should watch their posture as they lean towards swimmers, bending from the knees rather than leaning from the waist. It is also important for them to wear suitable comfortable clothing and shoes.

It is important to remember that even children, who seldom lose their voices, can be hoarse after a gala. This is because the noise rebounds off the hard surfaces and swimmers and supporters find themselves shouting louder and louder in order to hear themselves. All that those in the water hear is a roar of sound. It is in this highly competitive atmosphere that problems can occur. The usual advice about drinking large quantities of water applies here too, because pools are usually overheated. If possible, teachers who are not involved in the gala should be encouraged to keep discipline on the bus going back to school in order to prevent additional vocal damage.

The teacher as entertainer

Within this role the teacher may be expected to perform as the disc jockey at a noisy disco, call the dances at a fund-raising barn dance, make the public address announcements at fêtes, and perform, often unwillingly, at leavers' parties! Of all these activities the most vocally dangerous is to shout above the noise of the disco; a microphone should always be used in such instances. Teachers should try to avoid being forced into entertaining by offering to contribute in another way.

The teacher as actor/director

Within this role the untrained teacher may be expected to conduct the drama club, or even teach GCSE drama, produce a class or drama festival play or, in its most basic, but by no means simplest, form, read and tell stories to groups of younger pupils. Drama classes are, by their very nature, highly participatory and noisy, and should be controlled by means of a non-verbal signal, such as a tambourine.

Although the purpose of a drama class is to develop and encourage verbal communication between pupils, at best it also develops cooperative skills. By focusing on interpersonal communication and mutual support, the group can avoid the chaos that results from drama classes that simply expend energy. When a degree of ensemble work develops, the drama class works best and both pupils and teachers enjoy the experience. The inexperienced director would be advised to avoid taking on a full-length production in the primary school, because these tend to be too long for children to sustain an interest in, either as performers or as audience. Parents also find extra rehearsals and long evenings difficult if younger children are involved. Professional child actors are not allowed to be on stage for more than 2 hours – perhaps the same unwritten law should apply to school productions. It is also important to enlist parental and staff support with regard to organization and assistance, and to delegate from the outset. In primary schools the themed programme, rather than the full-scale play, allows participation from other departments such as music, art and gym, and provides involvement from a broad range of children, not just the best actors. Parents do not expect to see 'professional' standards in a school production and much of the charm lies in the unexpected 'hiccup'. As a general rule, a well-rehearsed shorter performance provides an experience that is better for the audience and more positive for the class, than an over-ambitious lengthy production.

The teacher as reader

Within this role the teacher may be expected to read aloud to the class. Most teachers read aloud well and enjoy doing so, but there are a significant number for whom this is a daunting and often vocally tiring task. There are those who 'feel the throat tighten' as they read and hear a voice produced that they find difficult to recognize as their own; others feel inhibited and self-conscious when having to entertain or be seen to be performing. The close link between 'theatre' and the classroom is recognized by many and for some it is an element that they really feel happy about. There are those who are natural communicators and there are those who feel that they did not enter teaching to be 'performers'.

Those teachers who are most likely to find themselves in the position of having to read to a class regularly are the pre-primary, infant and primary school teachers, in addition to teachers of English literature and other humanities subjects, and those whose duties include reading at assembly. Teachers of the younger age groups expect to read aloud regularly, but teachers who find themselves with a class that they did not originally train for are often worried about how effectively they can 'tell the story'. When there is anxiety over the reading the voice is likely to become overused and tired. Some Postgraduate Certificate of Education (PGCE)-trained teachers, who found themselves in a position of having to read aloud, have reported that their 1-year course did not provide the practice that they felt they needed to read as well as they would have wished to their class.

Teachers are all knowledgeable about the rudiments of reading and so there is no need to reiterate them here. That there is a significant difference between fluent personal reading and the art and skill of reading aloud to an audience is not often acknowledged. The most important of these differences is that the reader has the book in front of him or her and can follow the printed word, whereas the audience cannot. The audience therefore is at a considerable disadvantage, and must be helped to 'enter the world of the story'. The art of the teacher who reads to the class is the important art of the story-teller, and this, sadly, is an art that is being eroded and replaced by television and video. In the lives of many children, the primary school teacher is the only adult who ever reads to them. The classroom 'story' takes on enormous importance for children who are not lucky enough to be read to in the home. Most teachers want to read aloud to the best of their ability, because they want children to be stimulated and excited by words and language, and to be inspired to read avidly for themselves.

The following are some simple suggestions that could make a considerable difference to the ease and quality of reading aloud:

- Speech has to be heard, decoded and understood before the audience can react to it, so it is important to allow the audience time and space to go through the listening process. The speaker should share in the process of story-telling by engaging the children's imagination and formulating images of the language as they receive it.
- Younger children need to be close to the reader so as to participate in the two-way process of the story. But, whatever their age, where possible the class should be brought closer to the speaker to save the voice being overused. This will also improve the chances of reading *to* the group rather than *at* them. A percentage of children may have undetected hearing problems and, as lip-reading is an important component of the listening process, the children should be encouraged to look at the speaker. Both physical and audible information should be given, by allowing the face and the body to convey the story, e.g. through eye contact when appropriate. Clarity is enhanced by muscular shaping of the sounds of speech with the lips and tongue. When a reader is committed to the story and to the telling of it, these aspects generally fall into place.
- Even before you speak you are having some effect on the listeners. Whether this effect is positive or negative is dependent on the body language that you use. At best the body should be alert but relaxed because any unwanted excess tension will transfer itself to the voice, so make sure that your chair is comfortable and that you have a glass of water close at hand. The class, too, should be comfortable and should avoid slumping on to desks. Story-telling should be a two-way communication process with listening being as important as reading or speaking.
- As mentioned before, eye contact is needed in order to relate to the listeners. It also helps to phrase meaningfully and to emphasize specific, appropriate words, so as to keep the feeling that the story is being told, not just read. For some teachers making eye contact while reading is 'easier said than done'. The usual comment is that the teacher is afraid of losing the place, which can easily happen in text tightly packed on

to the page. When reading anything complicated, such as Dickens or even Mark Twain, the advice is to scan the chapter first and to become familiar with it. If the individual knows exactly what he or she is going to read and when, e.g. if having to read a religious extract at an assembly, the extract should be photocopied and if necessary enlarged. A highlighter should be used to mark words or phrases that can signal a pause or an opportunity for the reader to look up. Readers sometimes look up with alarming regularity because they have been led to believe that any eye contact represents good reading practice. They do not make eye contact with sincerity but rather flick their eyes over the listeners before returning hurriedly to the text. For the listeners, 'looking up' can be annoying if it is done without reason. The golden rule for readers is to look up only when it is appropriate and to be aware of the whole class, not just a section of it. Eye contact should allow the reader time to include the class and allow them time to digest what has just been said. Occasionally it may be appropriate to repeat a phrase or a word from the text in order to increase the level of the group's involvement, but it is important to remember that the class do not have the text in front of them, nor are they able to cast their eyes ahead and anticipate the story. The value for the class lies in being read to by an adult whom they know and can relate to; unless the reader makes contact with the class, they may as well have listened to the radio.

- Most people reading aloud read at a faster pace than they realize. Monitoring the speed at which an individual is reading or speaking is difficult, particularly if the individual is under pressure and does not naturally enjoy the delivery of words. The reader's greatest asset is the ability to give him- or herself and the audience time. The audience needs time to digest one idea before being fed another; they need to be able to hear how one idea develops into the next so that they can build up the progression of ideas and be involved in the development of the narrative. They also need time to 'take on board' new characters, often with unusual names, and to build up, from the language that they hear, a visual image of the action, as well as formulating a response to the incidents and emotions. A slower speech rate also helps the reader, because it allows for eye contact, changes of vocal tone for different characters and the building up of an imaginative response to the text and, if the reader does not know the story, it allows them to go through their own 'see, decode, understand and react' process.
- The ability to scan ahead is something that can be improved by practice and confidence. Often it is the panic of losing the place that prevents an otherwise confident sight-reader from letting the eyes glide over the page. A most useful exercise is to hold a closed book and open it suddenly; let the eyes fall on to a phrase; close the book; look up and speak the phrase. At first the eyes flicker frantically over the page and

have to be encouraged to settle on a phrase. If this is done regularly it builds ability and confidence, and is an excellent exercise to do with children from 9 years onwards. It begins to extend the eye's peripheral vision and it is this that allows the full sense of phrases to be taken in and choppy, broken reading improved. It is great fun and can be practised first using lists of phrases and idioms, because they are less daunting than great blocks of text. Progression can then be made on to more densely blocked text, using books that have larger writing and good spacing.

The teacher as tour guide

Within this role the teacher may be expected to conduct tours to museums, give information on the dinosaur while counting heads, or traipse across battlefields, battle against the wind and cold and project the voice, while describing the action. This role can also include skiing trips, sports tours and a week's educational field trip abroad. In these circumstances the teacher has to use the voice at high volume for long periods of time in adverse circumstances. As with the field sports teachers, it is important for the teacher to draw the group around him or her and so avoid having to project in the noise of, for example, a busy tourist centre. It is important for children to be encouraged always to position themselves in a semi-circle around the teacher so that they may see the teacher and the teacher may see them.

The teacher as music teacher

Within this role the teacher may be expected to be involved in singing classes. For men teaching singing in the primary school, problems can arise, because the teacher often has to sing at a pitch far higher than his natural one, which can be both problematic and 'tiring'. Male teachers sometimes have difficulty sustaining high pitch for long periods of time, especially those who work with junior schoolchildren or in girls' schools. The use of falsetto is one option but, if in attempting to reach high notes it creates vocal tension, it should be avoided. Instead the note may be suggested through the use of an instrument such as a recorder.

Singing and music teachers, if they are not aware of good positioning at the piano or while bending over seated children playing recorders, may experience postural problems. Alignment at the piano should be checked; teachers are advised to avoid standing and leaning over to play while at the same time looking up at the class and attempting to sing. This also applies to situations that involve playing while looking backwards at a class. If at all possible, the instrument should be positioned so that it may be used in the best possible physical position.

Teachers should try to 'practise what they preach'. If the class is being told how to breathe, teachers should make sure that they are taking time to breathe themselves. Children should be taught that the breath should be low and deep. Most children remember choir teachers saying 'Take a big breath' which invariably ends up being a breath that allows far less intake of breath than a breath taken low in the body, using the lower ribs, diaphragm and abdominal muscles. Shoulders should be relaxed; playing the piano and string instruments can be conducive to shoulder tension, e.g. the physical position for violinists can lead to a forward head and neck position and it is therefore important for this to be monitored. Many music teachers teach in the lunch break and it is important to make sure that, rather from rushing from one class into another, teachers take some time out for themselves. If demonstrating to the class, the teacher should not do so when suffering from a cold and, rather than speaking or singing over the noise of the class, the teacher should instead first signal for them to stop.

The teacher as counsellor in pastoral care

Within this role, the teacher may be expected to take part in parent evenings. For many teachers this is an extremely stressful occasion because it almost always follows on after a full day's teaching. Most parents, while concerned about their children, are appreciative of what is done by teachers and are generally good-natured, but occasionally they can be defensive or even aggressive. Although assaults are uncommon, the pressure on the teacher is enormous and the effect on an already tired and stressed individual is considerable.

The most vocally challenging situation for teachers is when more than one teacher shares the same space for consultations, because this increases the ambient noise level. This situation does, however, impose time limits which are strictly controlled to avoid some parents or carers taking up more than the allotted time.

To lessen the pressure on the teacher and protect the voice the following strategies are proposed:

- If possible make sure that there is time to have a proper break between the usual working day and the timetabled parent consultations.
- It is important for teachers to keep well hydrated throughout the evening. Ideally, tea breaks should be scheduled into an evening of consultations.

- Seating should be comfortable. Straining over the table while talking should be avoided. Head and shoulder position should be checked and monitored throughout the evening.
- It is important for teachers to be honest but polite to parents and not to allow themselves to become intimidated.
- Chairs should be well positioned so that there is no need for the teacher to raise his or her voice when talking to parents. The consultation should be planned so that opening and closing statements are available to signal clearly that the consultation is over. Possible phrases to use are: 'Well it's been good to talk to you/meet you, and I will contact you if the situation doesn't seem to improve' or 'Thank you for coming and please congratulate John on the effort he has made'.
- Standing up and offering a hand will also signal that the interview is over.

These are just some of the additional duties and requirements demanded of the teacher. Obviously some teachers are not going to become involved in all or any of these roles. In larger schools there are likely to be specialists in each area, but from time to time a teacher finds that a new job makes unusual demands or that in order to take promotion they will have to widen their field of activities. Teachers moving into head teacher posts or head of year posts are going to have to take on many of the duties mentioned.

In taking on these posts personality is a significant factor; not every teacher is willing to face the wider audience. They may feel happy to teach 15-year-old 'tearaways' but are daunted by their parents. Some teachers enter the profession because they enjoy the links between teaching and the public role. There is a large professional crossover between teachers and actors, and between teachers and people who originally considered entering the church. These careers share may necessary skills and personality qualities. There will, however, always be aspects of any job that an individual will dislike. Many teachers enjoy the performance element of teaching. Others love to teach but hate to perform and feel very strongly that, when they entered the profession, these peripheral demands were never made clear to them. Unfortunately, without the willingness to carry out at least some of these duties effectively, career prospects may be limited. One way of surmounting the problem is for teachers to remain resolute if asked to undertake a commitment that they do not feel able to handle, although this is not to under-estimate how difficult it can be to withstand persuasion.

The teacher in the role of supply teacher

'Supply' is a role that many teachers take on for a variety of reasons. Some teachers, returning to teaching after a period away, raising a family perhaps, choose not to return to full-time work immediately. Others may have moved from one area to another and may choose to experience a variety of schools in the new area before applying for a permanent post. Whatever the reason, there are a number of specific demands made on the teacher in this role.

The employment of supply teachers has increased enormously over recent years. They not only step into the breach when staff members are sick but also provide cover so that teachers have free time for administrative work and planning, and to allow for inset training. More frequently they fill the gaps that occur between permanent staff leaving and new appointments being made. It appears to be a workforce that is growing as stress in schools increases, resulting in absenteeism. As such they form an important section of the teaching community but one that at present receives little support or development in training.

Supply teachers encounter difficulties as a result of the variable nature of their work. They may be teachers who do not want a permanent position, or teachers who have found the administrative workload too much and want simply to be able to do what they were trained for and teach. There are a great number of supply teachers for whom working as a supply is a career choice. It would appear that a considerable number of supply teachers are immigrants to the UK, and many were not trained in the British teacher training system, nor have they previously taught in the country. For some English may be a second language. The same situation is undoubtedly the case for supply teachers in the USA and other countries.

It would be wrong to presume that all supply teachers will encounter problems; there will be many who have had years of successful teaching and whose training may have included a solid grounding in voice work, but for some this is not the case. Many highly experienced teachers from other countries have qualifications not recognized by British education authorities. These teachers may be working with unqualified status on lower salaries.

Problems encountered by supply teachers

The teacher who does not teach on a regular basis is less likely to build muscle stamina steadily over a number of weeks. This can be a problem for some working in supply especially when they suddenly encounter a noisy class or find themselves teaching a week of physical education.

Others actually find this sporadic pattern better for their voices, because they do not need to accept a job if their voice is tired.

A constantly changing challenge

A major cause of difficulty for supply teachers is that they are always entering an 'unknown zone'. They are constantly negotiating new student–teacher relationships as well as meeting new colleagues and being outsiders in an unknown situation. At times supply teachers are not properly met and introduced to colleagues or given essential information. There can be confusion as to which classes will be taught by the supply teacher, which leads to delays at the start of the class and in turn breaks the sense of 'normality' for the students. Some students see the supply teacher as an easy target and take the opportunity to 'have some fun' at their expense by swapping names or inventing them, when asked who they are. Others give incorrect directions as to the whereabouts of classes and other teachers, in order to confuse the supply teacher and make them late. Students have been known to state 'I don't do work for supply teachers' when asked to get on with their work.

Discipline can be difficult because the students know that the teacher will not be around for long, so they will probably not be challenged about their behaviour. This may result in the class becoming noisier than usual and the teacher using high volume or finding it necessary to shout. If the teacher works sporadically he or she may not have sufficient time to build vocal stamina and may therefore be more susceptible to vocal problems.

Common problems encountered by supply teachers

- Not all schools provide the supply teacher with enough information, such as clear directions to the school, maps of the layout of the school, catering facilities and toilets.
- Classrooms often lack adequate essential materials such as fresh and working felt-tip pens for the white boards.
- Sometimes instructions are not given clearly or correctly, so that the teacher may have prepared one lesson, and then have suddenly to change the content and work without proper preparation.
- Work set by the class teacher may not have been left out in a place where it is easily visible, leading to delay and a loss of class focus.
- The teacher may not be familiar with the subject at all – this can be particularly difficult when a subject requires specialized knowledge such as mathematics, a foreign language or science.

- Even if the supply teacher has previously taught the subject he or she may have to adapt to a very different way of approaching it. Help in doing so may not be easy to find because of pressure of work on the permanent staff.
- A complaint from supply teachers is that, as a result of poor organization on the part of the school, or bad behaviour in the class, they do not teach but 'care take'. This can be professionally frustrating.
- Supply teachers sometimes find themselves working with the same class for a longer period of time if the need arises. Although they are then able to bond with the class, some teachers find that the parents do not take them seriously, especially if the teacher needs to discipline the child.
- Supply teachers are by their very existence a 'second best' option. The class is always better catered for by a permanent teacher with shared experience and knowledge of the class. If a class is continuously being presented with temporary staff their work will suffer, and they know this and feel neglected. For many working in supply teaching, the system works best if the same teachers return regularly to the same school, so that they become an accepted member of the school community. This is not always possible.

All these pressures and confusions create tension and undoubtedly place demands on the posture, breath and confidence of the teacher. Other problems for the supply teacher are more personally specific:

- The teacher may not be local and may have to travel a considerable distance to get to the school. This may mean that the teacher is often tired especially if he or she has taught at several different schools in one week. The travel may have involved waiting in draughty bus stations or the teacher may arrive at school cold and then spend the day in the heated classroom. The teacher may leave home much earlier than is necessary in order to negotiate new routes and unknown distances.
- Agencies ring round teachers on their list once the need becomes apparent at the start of the school day. This means that teachers relying on supply work must be ready to teach every day, although they may not get work. Alternatively they may receive a late summons and be ill-prepared and have to rush around at the last moment arriving at the school tense and flustered.
- There are additional strains on the supply teacher, which may lead to an increased likelihood of vocal stress or ill-health. In primary schools supply teachers are expected to stay at school and mark the day's work before they leave. This can result in a very long day and can become a problem if the teacher works every day. The supply teacher meets a new set of students and a new set of 'germs' several times a week, so they may be more susceptible to infection.

- The teacher may be returning to teaching after a break and his or her confidence may be low. The effects of low self-esteem and a sense of not belonging may impact on posture and breath.
- The career supply teacher does not have a salary to rely on and is dependent on working as often as possible in order to earn a living. They know that they have long periods out of work during the school holidays and so are often reluctant to refuse work when it is offered. This means that they are more likely to teach when they are not well, and when they would take a day off if they were permanently employed.

The supply teacher is increasingly a crucial member of the teaching profession. The job is a difficult and demanding one and requires flexibility and confidence. As supply teachers are not on a school's permanent staff roll, it is often difficult for them to access ongoing training in order for them to respond to the changing curriculum and to serve the students as best they can.

The many different roles assumed by teachers are possible only because of their flexibility and ability to respond to the demands that the profession makes on them.

11 Practical work

Readers will note a change in the writing style in the two remaining chapters of the book. This has been done in order to address the reader directly in order to make the exercises more accessible and easier to follow.

This chapter offers a variety of exercises, which have a broad application to all voice users. Some will, by their nature, be more appropriate to class situations but many offer a firm foundation for general voice use. The exercises aim to establish an integrated physical and vocal approach. Some exercises are for specific muscles; others offer a planned sequence of exercises or routines for the voice. Regular periods of exercise are preferable to occasional long sessions and therefore these routines are designed to last for between 10 and 20 minutes. You may notice some repetition of exercises within different routines.

The exercises raise awareness of habitually held tension in muscles, establish low placement of the breath, and encourage efficient use of energy in body and voice. Habits of any sort are difficult to change and often develop out of the individual's personality and his or her reaction to situations, making it difficult for the individual to be objective about where and how tension is held, and so working with another person can be helpful. The way in which people like to work is also highly individual; in recognition of this, we have included a variety of approaches so that, if one approach does not appeal, another may. If the vocal problem is a recurring one, we would strongly advise seeking professional help before starting on an exercise plan. These exercises will help maintain a healthy voice and prevent problems caused by inappropriate breathing and physical alignment, but should never be seen as a substitute for voice therapy if that is required. The participative value of voice work within the classroom has already been stressed, so we have also included exercises that can be done with primary and secondary classes.

Posture exercises

1a. Stand as badly as you can (you can involve adolescent classes in this exercise) with the weight on one foot, not two, the ribs compressed, the arms folded across the body, the shoulders raised, the head and neck slumped forwards, and the spine curved. Notice how the eye level has fallen.

1b. Now move from this posture into a more balanced and open position with the weight over both feet; drop the arms to the sides, lengthen the spine, open the rib cage, lower the shoulders, and balance the head on the top of the spine.

Notice where the eye level is now. Do not over-correct.

1c. Repeat this exercise and when you begin to create the open posture do so by gradually 'internally' adjusting the posture by working through each vertebra individually, 'stacking' one on top of the other, and gradually sensing that there is greater length to the spine.

Try to 'sense' the muscles releasing and the body realigning. Avoid a sudden external correction.

2. Once you are in the balanced position with the knees relaxed and flexible, the pelvis level and not tilted either forwards or backwards, you can begin to stretch. Lift the arms above the head and stretch through the arms to the tips of the fingers while reaching for the ceiling. Look up at the ceiling while you stretch. Keep the feet on the floor and do not lose your balance. The stretch can be maintained for up to 30 seconds before you slowly lower your arms.

2a. As you begin the lowering process, allow the head to lower too. The weight of the head and shoulders will take the spine into a curve and the movement will eventually involve bending over at the waist and allowing the knees to bend until the body is completely bent over with the arms swinging loosely, touching the floor. Once in this position make sure that the head is free and allowed to hang loosely.

2b. Allow the jaw and tongue to be loose and free also. Gradually begin to uncurl, by building up one vertebra upon the next until the spine begins to unfold and lengthen. Leave the shoulders, head and neck until last. Once you are completely, but not rigidly upright, repeat the exercise a second and third time.

A word of caution: moving to an upright position too quickly can occasionally lead to a momentary feeling of dizziness, so uncurl the spine slowly.

Class exercise

Once you have established a sense of the free and open body ask the class to work in pairs. One of the pair should create different postures while the partner mirrors them. These postures may include well-aligned positions as well as slumped or over-corrected positions, weight badly distributed on one foot or hip, high shoulders or shoulders that are slumped and rounded, head jutting forward or pulled back. They should aim to finish on an open released posture. This allows the class to feel the differences between positive and negative postures and to observe the differences.

Shoulder exercises

1. Lift the shoulders up to the ears, hold this position for 5 seconds and then release. Repeat twice more.

2. Lift the shoulders in a shrug – making sure that they drop fully to a released position. This should be done several times a day.

3. Lift the shoulders up to the ears, then move them backwards so that the shoulder blades almost meet. Hold them in this position briefly, before releasing them and moving them forward and upward again. Continue the cycle for at least six rotations.

4. Raise the right arm above the head, stretching through the arm to the fingertips. Notice how the ribcage opens in this position. Take the arm backwards, breathing out as it descends and then complete the circle by lifting the arm up back to the starting point as breath flows back into the body. Repeat this exercise three times on the right side, taking care never to hold the breath, but noticing how the opened position of the ribs naturally draws breath in and that closing the ribs expels the air.

5. Repeat the same exercise with the left arm, making sure that you coordinate the breath with the action. (Breathe in as the arm is lifted and breathe out as the arm is lowered.)

Another useful exercise can be found in the routine for secondary schools later in this chapter.

Neck exercises

When working on the neck it is important to avoid fully rotating the head. Neck work should be gentle and should not place stress on the vertebrae. Extending the length of the neck should not be a forceful movement. Try to imagine that someone is gently brushing a hand up along the surface of the neck and 'think' the length of the neck rather than physically stretching it.

1. Beginning with the head in a balanced position, slowly drop the chin down on to the chest, feeling the extension of the muscles at the back of the neck. Do this three to six times, making sure that no movement is forced. Return the head to a balanced position and feel the length in the neck at the back.

2. Keeping the feeling of length in the back of the neck, but not over-extending it, take the head to the right shoulder and then, keeping the chin close to the chest, move the head slowly to the left shoulder. Repeat, starting at the left shoulder and moving towards the right one. Never rotate the head fully or do any neck exercises hurriedly.

3. Keeping the head balanced on the top of the spine, alternately lift and sway the shoulders up and down in a 'wave-like' motion. Keep the movement fluid and relaxed.

4. Using the image of the head balanced on a greasy ball-bearing at the top of the spine, allow the head to bob gently from the right shoulder to the left shoulder using gentle movements rather like those of a marionette.

Relaxation exercises

There are two very effective methods of relaxing on your own. The first is through a 'stretch and release' method and the second is through the use of image and the establishment of a feeling of release in the muscles that you are able to isolate. For most people, the tensions that they carry become habitual and are therefore difficult to isolate and to identify in specific muscles. Working to identify tension is the first step towards releasing it.

Stretching

1. Kneel on the floor, sit back on your heels and stretch the arms forward along the floor, so that you feel the stretch in the spine. Hold the stretch for a few seconds and then release it.

2. Lie on the floor with arms and legs in a star shape. Now stretch diagonally, so that the right arm and left leg are stretched away from the centre of the body. Hold then release. Then stretch the left arm and the right leg. Hold then release. Feel the sense of breadth in the back.

3. You can do this exercise either sitting in a chair or lying on the floor. If in a chair make sure that you are comfortable with sufficient support for your neck and lower back. If lying on the floor you may want to place a book under your head and bend your legs at the knee in order to reduce the curve in the lower back. In this exercise you issue instructions to yourself, beginning with the command to 'hold tension', then to release it and finally to assess the new muscle state. The aim of the exercise is to teach the body to differentiate between habitually held tension and the released state.

3a. Starting with the head, push it into the floor or the back of the chair. Hold the tension. Release the tension and then assess the different sensations in the muscles of the neck and those around them.

3b. Now push the shoulder girdle into the back of the chair or the floor. Give the self-instructed command 'hold'. After a few seconds self-instruct to 'release'. Then 'assess' the difference between the states of tension and release.

3c. Move on to the back. Push the spine into the floor or into the back of the chair. Hold the tension and then release and assess.

3d. Continue through the body, tightening and releasing buttocks, arms, fists, legs, feet, jaw and finally the whole body.

Image relaxation

Once more get comfortable either on a chair or on the floor. Make sure that you are warm. Think of a place you would like to be; imagine somewhere tranquil such as on a warm beach, in a field of flowers or on a gently rocking boat on a blue sea.

Use the image to create a feeling of peace. Imagine the feeling of the sun on your limbs. If possible play some relaxing music. Concentrate on the feeling that in this ideal setting you have no responsibilities or worries. Try to recreate the experience of being on holiday.

Now work through the body from the feet upwards, ensuring that each part of the body is relaxed. If you are not happy with the state of tension in a group of muscles, tighten the muscles in question and then release them. Work up slowly through the legs, pelvis and buttocks, spine, ribcage, chest, shoulders and arms, hands, fingers, neck, head and facial muscles.

Breathing exercises

1. Lie on the floor in a comfortable position with a small book under the head and the legs bent at the knee to avoid a severe curve in the lower back. Place a large book, or better still a brick, on the area of the diaphragm or just below the waistline. Relax either by doing one of the exercises in the relaxation section above, or by simply resting for a few minutes. Notice how, as you begin to relax and breathe from the area of the diaphragm, the action of the breath gently pushes the book or brick upwards as it enters the body and begins to fall as the breath leaves the body.

2. In this position the shoulders are not involved in the breathing process. As you breathe out allow the air to leave the body on a gentle /fff/. Once the air has left the body wait for the body to 'need' a new breath before taking one; if you over-breathe you will feel dizzy. It is important to breathe out at a slower speed than you breathe in. Notice how a rhythm develops. The breath comes in to a count of three or four, there is a slight pause and the breath leaves to a count of four or five. There should also be a pause before the new breath is inhaled.

3. Lying on your stomach, get your head into a comfortable position; most people find lying with the face to one side is best. Place the book or brick on to the buttocks, so that you can feel it rise and fall as you breathe in and out. This is a useful exercise because it allows you to feel the breath in a way that is impossible when you stand up, because you are lying on the abdomen and the action of the diaphragm when breathing in causes displacement of the internal abdominal organs. You are able to feel this as movement in the lower back and buttocks. It is also good for creating a feeling of 'separation' in the lower vertebrae, and allowing relaxation in muscles in an area that many of us hold in a state of tension.

4. Standing in front of a mirror, place one hand on the midriff. As you breathe out, place some pressure on the midriff and notice how the outgoing breath results in the muscles below the hand moving towards the spine. As breath comes into the body the hand will follow the muscles of the midriff outwards. While you are doing this, check in the mirror that the shoulders are not lifting significantly as breath comes in. Begin to develop a more conscious outward breath using /fff/ to the count of five. Pause and then feel the breath come in under the hand to the count of three, followed by /fff/ out to the count of five. Once confident with these exercises, increase the duration of the outgoing breath from five to seven or eight. Never force this; what is important is that you become conscious of the fact that the body expands as breath comes in and decreases in size as breath is exhaled.

5. Stand with your hands stretched outwards in a star position. Breathe out on an /s/ and as you do so bend over to touch the floor, allowing your knees to bend as you go over. Pause until you feel the need to breathe. When you do, stand up and return to your original position and feel the breath re-entering the body as you do so. The object of this exercise is to illustrate that the open body position produces an effortless intake of breath and, when the ribcage is not constricted, breath freely enters the body. This illustrates that a good open posture is a very important aid to good breathing.

Are you a breath-holder?

For some teachers the problem is associated more with learning to release breath than with learning to breathe in. We often stop ourselves breathing out fully and subsequently create a shallow in-breath.

Exercises for releasing held breath

The fight-or-flight/flee response has been examined in an earlier chapter. When we are under stress of any sort, a common reaction is to lock the neck and shoulders and hold the breath. Many teachers are familiar with the physical feeling of being 'locked' that results from a degree of panic. The resultant 'fixing' of the head and neck prevents the body being able naturally to exchange incoming and outgoing air. This means that the mind and body are unable to benefit from the subsequent calming effect of this action. When we hold breath or 'fix' the head and neck, we immediately become 'bound' and lose our ability to be responsive to the world around us. We are usually very aware of the need to take breath in, in order to prepare for speech, but often do not release the breath as we speak, resulting in a sound that is not breath supported. The advice to 'breathe out' when under pressure may seem very simplistic but it is very helpful. With the outgoing breath, many held tensions are released.

Here are some exercises that will ensure that you stop holding and fixing. Most of them can be done anywhere. To begin with use a voiceless 'sound' such as /ff/, /ss/, /sh/, /th/ and feel the breath pass over the tongue or lips as it is released.

1.   Raise and drop the shoulders releasing the breath as you let the shoulders fall.

2.   Sigh out deliberately and noisily, expelling breath not voice.

3.   Stretch up to the ceiling and then collapse from the waist, releasing the breath as you do so.

4.   Imagine that you need to push a car up a hill. As you prepare for the action the breath fills the lungs; as you 'push' you will notice that you contain the breath within the lungs (the ribcage remains open.) Once you have completed the action and reached your goal and relax, you will notice how the surplus breath leaves the lungs. Repeat several times noticing the preparation, holding and release of the breath.

5.   Standing with feet wide apart stretch arms out to the side and lengthen the spine and neck, making the body as broad and as long as possible. Hold the position for a few seconds and then release the arms. Notice that the breath, which has been held, is also released. Avoid shortening the spine by slumping.

6.   Now repeat the previous body position and this time make sure that you do not hold the breath, but actively free the neck and abdominal muscles and breathe in and out freely while keeping the spinal length.

7.   Imagine that you are eager to speak but as soon as you are about to begin someone else speaks first. Notice the momentary holding of breath each time you are interrupted.

8. Imagine that you are blowing the petals off a dandelion. A long sustained breath is best. Try blowing five short sharp blasts of breath to remove all the petals from the dandelion. Make sure that your breath action comes from the centre of the body.

9. Imagine that you are bouncing a ball using one hand. As you bounce the ball release the breath on /pah/. Then experiment by holding your hand to your mouth and feel the breath on your hand.

10. Using your arm as a scythe, engage the breath to produce the sound /fff/ as you 'slice through long grass'. Begin with one 'slice' on one breath and build to four separate 'slices' on one breath.

11. Imagine that you are performing a martial art and 'punch and slice' the air releasing breath as you do so. Explore different qualities of breath on /fff/, /sh/, /woo/, /kkk/ as you move.

12. Using an imaginary ball, roll it across the floor on a smooth soundless stream of breath. 'Follow it' to its destination with both the arm and the breath. Repeat using /fff/, /sss/, /mah/, /moo/.

13. Holding your hand up to your mouth release a thin stream of breath on to your hand silently. Then with a wide-open throat, breathe all your breath SILENTLY through an open throat and mouth on to your hand. You should feel the broad column of warm air but hear no sound at all. If you hear a rasping noise, there is tension in the throat. Make sure that you 'feed' the breath through from the low centre of the abdomen.

Having done these exercises you should have experienced what it feels like to hold on to breath and release it. Once you can identify the sensation, you are well on the way to learning to release it. Try to catch yourself holding your breath. If you do, make sure that you release your shoulders, neck and jaw and actively breathe out. If the occipital joint at the base of the skull and the top of the spine is locked, free exchange of breath is unlikely so it is important to work on the neck exercises in order to free this point.

Jaw exercises

The mouth is the only truly moveable resonator and it is important for it to be relaxed and flexible in order for voice and speech to be resonant and free. Any releasing exercises should be done from the 'hinge' of the jaw and not from the front of the mouth.

1.   Yawning is an excellent way to release tension in the jaw and pharynx, and the release of tension increases muscularity. Do not stifle yawns; enjoy them.

2.   Imagine that you are chewing a piece of toffee. Use the whole mouth space and jaw. To avoid this becoming a way of inadvertently increasing tension in the jaw, work with a relaxed, almost slow motion energy that aims to stretch the strap muscles of the jaw.

3.   Imagine that you have small springs between your molars, which do not allow your teeth to touch, so that the result of attempting to bring the teeth together would be that they spring away from each other. This springing movement also increases the length of the jaw muscles.

4.   Place your hands on either side of the face and gently stroke the jaw downwards. Allow the mouth to open as the hands move down the face. Keep the jaw loose, free and mobile.

5.   Holding on to the chin with the thumb and fingers of one hand, tip the head backwards, as if you were able to lift the upper jaw. Create space in the mouth and between the teeth. Keep the tongue relaxed.

Exercises for the articulators

1.   Lips need to be exercised in order to keep the muscles capable of making firm explosive sounds flexibly and without creating neck and jaw tension. First, purse the lips forward and then spread them suddenly into a broad smile. It is important to be aware of the muscles used in the two activities.

2.   Curl the upper lip up towards the nose. Curl the lower lip down towards the chin. Purse the lips and then open and close the pursed lips in an action that resembles the mouth of a goldfish.

3.   Try balancing a pencil on the upper lip.

4. Blow up the cheeks and then using your fingers 'pop' the cheeks, producing a sound as the air explodes through the lips.

5. Produce an exploding /b/ sound using the lips. Increase this to three /b/s followed by a vowel, e.g. /b/b/bah/. Do the same with /p/ and /p/p/pah/. Follow this with vowels that end on a /b/, e.g. /oob/ and /ohb/, and with /p/, e.g. /oop/ and /ohp/.

6. The tongue needs to be exercised so that it is capable of flexible movement without tension. To start, simply stretch the tongue as far out of the mouth as you can and then allow it to relax back into the mouth, leaving the tip touching the lower front teeth.

7. The following exercise aims to stretch the middle of the tongue. Place the tip behind the lower front teeth and then bunch the middle of the tongue forward and out of the mouth. Hold the stretched position for a few seconds and then release.

8. Lift the tongue to the ridge behind the upper teeth and explode the consonant sequence /d/d/d/d/ and /t/t/t/t/. Lift the tongue and form an /l/, then precede the /l/ by a series of vowels, e.g. /eel/, /ool/, /ahl/, /ohl/, /awl/. Use a series of words containing /l/ to exercise the tongue; these can be done with children, asking them to supply the words, e.g. lorry, land, light, cool, feel, hold, golden, lazy, languid.

Routines

Routine 1: floor exercises

1. *Spine*: lengthen the spine. Imagine that you are able gently to separate the vertebrae by moving the head away from the shoulders and the hips from the ribs. Broaden the back by imagining that you can widen the shoulder girdle. Gently press the shoulders into the floor, then release. Feel that you are longer and broader than you were.

2. *Jaw and tongue*: imagine that the jaw hangs off the skull. Feel the space between the teeth. Stretch the tongue out of the mouth, release it and allow it to slip back to a position where it loosely touches the front teeth. Clench the teeth, release and then release a second time. Repeat the exercise three times.

3. *Scalp*: release the muscles of the face and scalp. Imagine that you are wearing a tennis sweatband across the forehead. Using the muscles of the face and head, imagine pushing it off the top of the head.

4. *Neck*: release the back of the neck by lengthening it. It sometimes helps to push the head gently into the floor; feel the tension, then release it. Gently move the head from the left to the right shoulder. Bring the head back to a central position.

5a. *Breath*: place one hand on the centre of the body, in the region of the navel. The most extensive breathing activity should ideally happen below the sternum and in the area of the abdomen and lower ribs. At best, the movement you feel as the breath displaces the muscles of the abdomen should be below the navel. Sigh out a feeling of being bored. Notice how the breath returns on its own. Sigh out a feeling of relief; again notice how the breath returns on its own.

5b. Breathing out, notice how the hand sinks down towards the floor. Feel the breath pass over the lips on a gentle /fff/. When you have emptied the lungs, pause and wait until you feel the need for breath. Do not resist it, simply allow the breath to return and notice how the hand on the body rises up towards the ceiling and the lower ribs move upwards and outwards to allow the breath to fill the space below the sternum. The shoulders, neck and upper chest need not be involved.

5c. Repeat the exercise above breathing out on the sound /sh/. Notice that the breath is used up more quickly on this sound.

5d. In your head, count to five on an /s/ as you breathe out. Make sure that you keep the neck and jaw loose. Do not worry about the quality of the /s/. On the next outgoing breath count in your head to six, and so on. Do not feel that it is important to reach a high number. If you get tense and tight in attempting to do so you have defeated the object of the exercise. Notice that the ribs as well as the muscles under the hand are active in releasing the breath.

5e. Now feeling very loose (the idea of being pleasantly drunk helps) turn the outgoing breath into sound and voice the sound /mah/. Build a feeling of vibration in the 'mask' of the face on /mmm/ before opening on to the vowel.

5f. Do the same using /nah/, /vah/ and /zah/.

5g. Begin to vary both the pitch and the vowel so that you produce a combination of sounds beginning with /n/, e.g. /noh/, /naw/, /nay/, /now/; do the same using /v/ and /z/.

Routine 2: working in a chair

1. Begin by sitting in an upright chair (such as one commonly used in class-rooms). Make sure that you find it comfortable. Sit with both 'sitting bones' firmly on the seat. Avoid sitting on one buttock only. Lengthen the spine from the coccyx to the skull. Avoid over-correction and hollowing of the lower back. Feel that the spine is free and flexible. Use the Alexander Technique image of a water fountain spouting up through the spine. Let the head be balanced on the top of the spine. Make small movements to the muscles of the neck so as to move the head minimally. No large movements of the head should occur. The feeling to work for is that of the marionette's head, loose but not floppy. Let the jaw feel as if it 'hangs off' the head. Let the tongue feel loose and free in the mouth with the tongue tip touching the lower front teeth.

2. Take the chair and sit back to front on it, so that you can lean over the backrest. This will open up the vertebrae in the lower spine and, as long as you release and 'let go' of the shoulders, it is a good position for breathing. You can put your head on your folded arms across the back of the chair.

3. If possible, ask someone to place his or her thumbs on your spine with the fingers splayed around the lower ribs. This will allow both of you to feel the expansion of the ribs when you breathe in. The movement will result in the thumbs moving away from the spine.

4. Set up a steady rhythm of breathing in and out. Work on breathing in to a count of three and then out to three, then in to a count of three and out to four, and in to three and out to five. As the breath leaves the body, feel it pass between the teeth and lips in a gentle /fff/. Never get competitive and try to get up to a high count, because this leads to breath-holding and creates more tension than it releases.

5. On the outgoing breath begin to introduce an effortless /vv/ by simply turning the breathed /fff/ into sound. Feel the vibrations on the lips and teeth and in the mask of the face. If you feel discomfort in the larynx or tension in the back of the neck, you are working too hard.

Resonance exercises

We recommend that work on 'opening up' the pharynx is done in conjunction with jaw exercises, so start by trying the following exercises.

1. Keep the lips together with light contact and then try to produce a full yawn or even an attempted or half-yawn.

2. Try to imagine chewing gum or toffee which increases in size with every chewing movement. As you do this you will be aware of the increased size and openness of the pharynx.

3. Try an 'inside' smile. In this exercise you relax the lips and 'smile' with the back of the mouth in the area of the oropharynx or where you feel the tonsils might be. The inside smile will increase your awareness of this area and encourage you to open it up. Some people find it easier to think of being an opera singer attempting to hit a very high note. Take up the posture of the effort but do not make any sound. This will give a sense of the placement of the inside smile.

4. Stick your tongue out as far as possible and then try to speak as clearly as possible with your tongue sticking out of your mouth. This is quite difficult to do but you can achieve a certain amount of clarity. It is fun to do and should not be taken seriously. If you use too much effort you may create more tension than you release, and you may 'gag' or your speech may sound nasal. These exercises often result in a need to yawn.

5. Try to create tension deliberately in the jaw, tongue and pharynx and speak a sentence in this very tight nasal way. It is useful to contrast the sound and sensation that you have when speaking in this manner with the sound and sensation that you have when the sentence is spoken without tension.

6. Contrast the full mellow sound that you achieve with an open relaxed pharynx with that of a tight constricted pharynx which results in a harsh metallic sound

7. Try to say the sentence 'Eve ate apples all afternoon' with excessively tight cheek muscles; then try it with excessively loose cheek muscles. Try the same sentence with a tight pulled-back tongue; now try it with a forward floppy tongue and finally try the same sentence with a tight clenched jaw and an excessively open one. Monitor the difference in tension in your cheeks, tongue and jaw in the production of these sentences. Also notice that the quality of the voice is altered when levels of tension change.

8. You can try the same combination of movements with these sentences:

   The five parked cars are mine.

   Now I see the fleecy clouds.

   Not hot rolled gold.

   Mark Parker sent a letter to settle the bet.

   Owen ought to go to Orlando.

   Exercises for the pharynx to develop increased pharyngeal resonance are very useful, not only in altering the resonance of the voice by finding a connection with the chest, but also in releasing areas of tension in the jaw and tongue.

9. Try to open your mouth as wide as possible and move into a yawn, feeling the increased space between the molars. Try to concentrate on increasing the space at the back rather than the front of the mouth, because if you try too hard to increase space at the front you will create some unwanted tension.

10. From the yawn move into a sigh as you breathe out. Use /ah/ or /aw/ for practice because this will encourage space in the mouth as well as in the pharynx. Your tongue tip should be touching the lower front teeth but should not be pressed against them.

11. Once you have established the yawn, try to sigh out on /oh/ and then say the following sentences keeping the pharynx as relaxed as possible.

   'I'd only own a gold opal', said Owen.

   Over and over and over again.

There is room for improvisation here and students can help by making up sentences as well. Working on the nasal resonators is more difficult because there is less 'room for manoeuvre' here. Some teachers will speak with regional accents that make greater or lesser use of nasal resonance. The importance of working on nasal resonance is to achieve a balance of oral, nasal and pharyngeal resonance.

12. Try the following sounds in sequence:

/ng ah/ /ng ah/ /ng oh/ /ng oh/ /ng ee/ /ng ee/

Make sure there is a contrast between the nasal /ng/ and the vowel so that the vowel remains clear and de-nasalized.

13. Try the following sentences, feeling the vibrations produced by the nasal resonance of the nasalized /m/ and /n/ sounds and the open oral resonance of the vowels.

My mother makes marvellous macaroni.

Mavis and Mildred munched on mackerel.

Many more men marry.

Musicians make music merrily.

Nora is a noisy nanny goat.

No naughty children are known here.

Routines

Routine 3: exercises in connecting resonators

(To be done after Routine 1 or 2, or after doing the resonance exercises.)

Sliding and gliding

Use the whole body and move whenever possible during these exercises.

1. *Sirening*: using the sound /n/ (and imitating the noise of a police siren) describe a vocal circle that begins between the shoulder blades and 'slide' the sound over the top of the head and face. Keeping the sound moving, return to the starting point along an imaginary circular trajectory. This should be easy as long as you keep it playful and do not try to push. You will not hurt the voice in this way. The same can be done with the /ng/ sound (in song) and the /m/, /v/ and /z/.

2. *Slide*: stretching up with hands in the air, allow the spine to bend over, one vertebra at a time, until you are bent over at the waist. As you do so make the sound of a vowel, such as /oo/, /ay/, /aw/ or /ah/. Make the vowel last as long as the journey from the extended stretch to the bent spine. This exercise can be done in reverse, starting the sound on the floor and sliding it upwards. Some people find this direction easier; others find it more difficult. Eventually both will be possible. If you find the onset of the vowel difficult precede it with an /m/.

3. *Bowling*: using the arm to bowl, imagine the ball is the sound /m/ and as it leaves your hand lift the sound up and over the space almost in an arc. Open to the vowel /ah/ halfway through the arc and sustain the sound until it 'lands' on the ground. Do this in slow motion so that it blends from the /m/ into the /ah/ smoothly as it arcs through the air.

4a. *Glide from chest to mouth*: make an /ah/ producing chest resonance. Feel the vibration by placing your hand on your chest. Make an /aw/ being aware of the resonance in the mouth. Notice how the lips form a megaphone shape.

4b. Begin by patting the chest while sounding /mah/ – feel the vibrations. Glide the /ah/ vowel into an /aw/ in the mouth, slurring from one sound to another, e.g. /mah . . . aw/

4c. Repeat the exercise beginning with the /aw/ resonating in the mouth and then glide this sound upwards into an /ee/. The glide from the /aw/ to the /ee/ should be relaxed and effortless, and the overall balance of one sound moving from one space to another should be maintained. In all these exercises the smooth continuum of sound is worked for and any feeling of pushed or strangulated sounds should be avoided. If a 'crack' in the flow of sound develops, just go slowly back over that area in the range. Using the hand or arm to describe the movement is often an effective aid to developing flexibility of the voice.

5. *Fire engine/ambulance siren*: using /ng . . . ah/ /ng . . . ah/ /ng . . . ah/, create the movement between head and chest resonance. This exercise explores the vocal range and extends the extremes of pitch and resonance. The dual-pitch siren is used for different vehicles in different cities, so the title of this exercise may not be correct for everyone, but can be adapted.

6. *Slurring and singing*: using a piece of text (just a few lines), slur the voice drunkenly and smoothly through the whole range. Try a line sung to a made-up tune. Speak it to that tune. Reduce the tune but keep the movement in the voice.

    It is important to 'play' and not to strive for perfection because this usually results in creating tension rather than releasing it.

Exercises for onset of the note

The term 'onset' refers to the approximation of the vocal folds in order to produce sound. The following exercises use /h/ before vowels because during the production of an /h/ the vocal folds do not come together completely and so limit hard attack.

Try using the following word list to achieve a gentle onset of the note. Use /h/ initially to achieve this, and then try the word without /h/.

h ...	*at*	*at*		*h ...*	*unusual*	*unusual*
h ...	*it*	*it*		*h ...*	*under*	*under*
h ...	*eat*	*eat*		*h ...*	*above*	*above*
h ...	*only*	*only*		*h ...*	*every*	*every*
h ...	*ill*	*ill*		*h ...*	*arm*	*arm*

Again it is very worthwhile to encourage your class to join in with these exercises; they can think of word lists as well as short sentences beginning with vowels, e.g.

Amy ate an apple.

Arnold's uncle urged him to eat up.

Esther owned an enormous elephant.

'All right Arthur move along immediately.'

In the second part of the exercise contrast it with the gentler onset experienced when beginning a word with an /h/:

Happy birthday Harriet.

How are you?

Here's a helping of ham.

Have some angel cake.

Exercises for teacher and pupils

1. Ask the class to stretch and yawn like a cat, not forgetting to stretch the spine, fingers and toes.

2. Everyone should wrinkle up the face so as to pull the ugliest face possible. Relax. Then smile as widely as possible. Relax.

3. Stretch the tongue out as far as possible as if 'pulling tongues'. Relax.

4. Blow through the lips like a horse in order to loosen the mouth area. Relax.

5. Imagine the class is playing tennis. To begin with, use the sound /b/ as the ball and everyone uses an imaginary tennis racquet to hit the /b/. The first part of the exercise is bouncing the /b/ on the racquet using short staccato sounds. The second part of the exercise is to lengthen the stroke so that the /b/ develops into a /bah/ and travels a distance. The distance should be specified, e.g. 'Let the /bah/ land on the floor at the other end of the line/classroom/hall'. Sometimes these exercises are best done in slow motion. The consonant /d/ can be similarly used and developed into /dah/ for the second part of the exercise.

6. If possible teach the class a nursery rhyme or a few phrases in a foreign language, so as to allow them to take up vocal and verbal positions not encountered in English or in the mother tongue.

7. Use 'mirroring' exercises in pairs to warm up the muscles of the face and the tongue. This requires the pair to work together and to focus on the specific muscles of speech. It is also fun and breaks down barriers.

Exercises for secondary classes

Exercises for teacher and pupils

1. Standing, ask the class to follow you in stretching up through the right-hand side. Take the arm above the head and over to the left side. The greatest extension is felt when the heel of the hand is used in the stretch. Now do the same with the left arm taking it up and then over to the right. Make the class aware of the movement of the ribcage in the stretch.

2. Ask the class to stand as badly as they possibly can. This usually involves standing with the weight on one leg, and the head and shoulders slumping forward. Often the arms will be folded across the chest and generally there will be a reduction of space between the hips and lower ribs, making easy breathing, centred in the diaphragmatic and lower rib area, difficult.

2a. The second part of this exercise is to ask them to correct the posture, so that they draw themselves up and out of the slumped position, readjusting their weight so that it is equally distributed across both feet. The spine will be long, the chest open and the head easily balanced on top of the spine. Once the class recognize the difference between 'bad' and 'good' alignment, they can take it in turns to stand badly so that a partner can physically change their posture by moving them into a more open and more aligned position. This exercise can be done as 'puppets' with quite young children, e.g. A is the puppet, B the puppeteer who rearranges the puppet's posture.

3. The class should now divide into pairs, and take it in turns to do the following exercises. One of the pair monitors and feeds back information to the partner actively involved in the exercise, a very important task. Feedback should be about the physicality observed and the level of tension monitored. Partner A stands in front of partner B and tries to release all tension from the shoulder area. Partner B then lifts the shoulder girdle of A and reports on how much, if any, resistance is encountered. Generally A will either hold the shoulders down or assist in raising them. The aim is to do neither, but rather to release the shoulders so that they can be moved by B. This is best achieved by attempting to isolate the shoulders and giving up all control over them. If the shoulders are locked they will be difficult to move; if, however, A is successful in isolating them, B will feel that they are heavy but loose. Feedback is very useful here because it begins to raise awareness of just how much tension is being held in the shoulder girdle. Change over so that A becomes the monitor and B does the exercise.

4. Once the shoulders have been released, a similar exercise is done with the arms. Partner A stands or sits with the arms hanging loosely by the sides. B lifts A's arm as A attempts to release the muscles, making the arm fully pliable and flexible and under the control of B. The temptation again is for A to control the arm, particularly when the arm is raised. When the arm is dropped by B, the arm may remain in 'mid-air', illustrating that the muscles retain tension. Change over and repeat, remembering the importance of feedback. The difficulty of releasing habitually held tension in the shoulders and the arms should not be under-estimated but this exercise is fun.

5. The class should stand, with knees unlocked and spine long. They should become aware of the way in which the head balances on the top of the spine and, releasing the jaw, should gently allow the head to nod in a small 'yes' gesture (up and down) and then in a 'no' gesture from side to side. Movements should be loose but minimal.

6. Move the head towards the right shoulder and, using the nose as a pencil, 'draw' straight lines from floor to ceiling, while travelling towards the left shoulder. The action here should again be one of fluidity and ease rather than of high energy. The muscles of the neck will feel the lengthening effect of the exercise. It is very important that the jaw should not be clenched.

7. In pairs again, A should stand in front of B. B places his or her hands around the lower ribs of A with the thumbs resting on either side of the spine. Beginning with A breathing out, B should notice how much the lower ribs decrease in width as breath is exhaled. The A group should be told to wait gently until they feel the need to breathe and then both A and B should notice how the breath replenishes and how, as it does so, B's hands on A's ribs move outward and the thumbs move away from the spine. Repeat, changing over A and B. it is important for B to feed back information about the movement as it occurs.

8. Ask the whole class to pat their chests as they release the sound /mah/. They should be encouraged to feel the vibrations in the chest. Imagine the class are drawing the letter /m/. They should use the hand slowly to describe the letter as the voice follows, thereby opening up and exploring the range. They can then describe a circle using /nnnnnnn/ while drawing the circle at the same time. In all these exercises it is important to feel the vibrations rather than listening to the sound.

9. Blow up the cheeks and with the fingers pop them. Blow raspberries. Make the noise of a motorbike to the sound /brmmmm/ and of a speedboat to the sound /vrmmmm/.

10. Using gibberish, ask members of the class to improvise a few lines in a made-up language and let the class repeat it. The object here is not to produce perfect sounds, but to explore a different usage of sound sequences.

11. Select a short passage of text that has energized language and let the class explore this together. Do not worry about analysing meaning; simply encourage exploration and enjoyment in the speaking of the words. Meaning will gradually evolve.

A quick warm-up

This warm-up uses some of the exercises already described in this chapter. Some warming up can be done quite inconspicuously in the bus or the car, or on the train.

Loosening the body

- Gently push the shoulder blades together and feel the opening of the front of the chest as you do so. Do this three times.

- Lift the shoulders slightly and then release them. Do this three or four times.

- Using two fingers of the right hand gently push the chin into the neck and feel the stretch of the muscles down the back of the neck. Do this three times.

- Imagine that the head is balanced on the top of the spine on a greasy ball-bearing.

- Move the head very smoothly and easily in a nodding 'Yes' motion.

Loosening the jaw

Checking the level of tension in the jaw is always recommended.

- Take the hands up to the cheekbones and gently stroke the jaw downwards allowing the strap muscle to release and lengthen.

- Imagine that the jaw is heavy and let its weight carry the jaw downward. Feel the separation of the teeth. Monitor whether or not the teeth are clenched; if so release the strap muscle.

Breathing out

- Sigh out to the count of five on an /ff/. When you finish the breath in the lungs simply allow them to refill.

- Sigh out to a count of six on an /ss/. Repeat the refill process.

- Sigh out to a count of seven on a /th/. Repeat the refill process.

- Sigh out to a count of eight on a /sh/. Repeat the refill process.

If you are in a private space (the car is ideal, as long as it is not overheated and your shoulders and neck are not locked in a state of tension as a result of traffic jams) you can begin to voice on the outgoing sigh.

- Sing out to a count of seven on /mmmmm/.

- Sing out to a count of eight on /vvvvv/.

- Sing out to a count of nine on /zzzzz/.

Always be aware of tension in the muscles of the neck when you sound, particularly as you come to the end of the breath capacity.

Moving the voice

- Describe a line from the floor to the ceiling using a trilled /r/. At first you may find that you cannot sustain the line of breath and sound but with practice you soon will.

Vowels

It is important to explore the length of vowels, e.g. /heat/, /he/ and /heal/ all contain the same vowel /ee/ but, depending on the sound that follows, the length of the vowel is altered.

- Try this sequence: /mmmm aw/ /mmmm oh/ /mmmm ee/, sustaining the vowel.

- Feel that the /mmm/ brings the voice forward on to the lips and that the vowels are free, forward and not held in the throat.

- Try working with /h/ in front of the vowels, e.g. /h-ah/ /h-ay/ h-aw/.

Lips and tongue

- Purse the lips and then circle them: beginning at the right-hand corner of your mouth, take the lips down to your chin, round to the left-hand corner and then up to the nose and back to the starting point. Reverse the action.

- Repeat the same exercise with the tongue and make sure that you stretch it and attempt to describe the full circle. Avoid missing out any section of the circle.

Consonants

When exercising the consonants it is important to feel the muscularity of the sounds, e.g. /b/ is made with a firm coming together of the lips and then exploded by the breath; /d/ is made by the lifting of the tongue to the teeth ridge and then being exploded by the breath; /f/ is made by the placing of the top teeth lightly on the lower lip and the fricative action of the breath as it passes through. The best way to exercise these sounds is to speak a short passage of verse that includes a plethora of consonants, e.g.

> *Full fathom five thy father lies,*
> *Of his bones are coral made;*
> *Those are the pearls that were his eyes;*
> *Nothing of him that doth fade,*
> *But doth suffer a sea-change*
> *Into something rich and strange.*

The Tempest by William Shakespeare (Act 1, scene 1)

12 Suggestions for volume, clarity and distance

For a significant number of teachers or lecturers, producing volume is a problem. If you cannot be heard your status is immediately undermined. In an attempt to create volume many teachers opt for what they consider the obvious solution – they shout – badly. The head thrusts forward and instead of creating more sound the voice becomes locked and strangulated. Those teachers with naturally soft voices may find themselves not necessarily shouting but 'pushing and squeezing' the voice out. This results in a hard, thin tone, which may be perceived as unfriendly, terrified, tentative or ungenerous. The effort involved in pushing the sound out is the very thing that limits it.

It is important to understand that in order to amplify sound what is needed is space for amplification, breath to carry the sound and placement of the voice at the front of the mask of the face. The fear involved in addressing large groups of people is likely to restrict these requisites and so a vicious circle can be created. It is often better to address such issues before attempting to approach them technically, but sometimes working on volume helps to overcome the fear by altering the relationship between the teacher and the class.

This chapter includes strategies that proved very useful in our workshops with teachers and that deal with commonplace activities undertaken by teachers. The first is the need to summon children from a distance or to address students who may be some distance from them. This often leads to the teacher thrusting the head forward and constricting the voice. The second strategy is for healthy 'shouting', which is an activity that many teachers find vocally difficult. The third is simply the need to use consonants and syllables in order to be clearly understood when addressing a large group.

We have spoken at length about the importance of posture and head position, and the freedom needed in the muscles of the neck and jaw. The instinctive energies rallied in situations requiring organization of large groups and involving any element of crowd control or discipline all work against the idea of the free neck. Many teachers find themselves using pointing and prodding gestures with the fingers and head and, when this happens, it is no surprise that not only the power in the voice is lost, but the control of the class goes too.

The value of stillness cannot be emphasized enough (by stillness we mean free, grounded stillness, not rigid, held stillness), not simply the stillness of the individual in the organizational position, but also the quietness and stillness required to allow breathing and thinking, and therefore learning, to take place. Status afforded to those who find a quality of quiet still control is generally high, and far outweighs that of teachers who expend a great deal of energy in order to achieve the same effect.

There are many misconceptions about making the voice easily audible. Most of these have evolved because the language used to encourage better audibility tends to produce an image of the voice 'pushing' forward. We hear 'Speak up', 'Speak out', 'Throw the voice', 'Project the voice', 'Reach the back of the room', 'Notch up the volume', and even 'Hit them with the sound'. In reality such suggestions only add to the teacher's tension through a misuse of energy. How much better, and of course more appropriate, it would be to suggest that the teacher 'Includes the whole class in the conversation' or 'Shares the information', so concentrating on the intention behind the word and conveying this intention, rather than simply creating more sound.

Some pointers from actors

Actors, often excellent communicators off stage as well as on, are not limited to high volume in order to be heard. When an actor is comfortable in a very large space, he or she is able to reduce volume to the minimum without losing clarity. They have learned how effectively resonance gives body and carrying power to the voice, and how keeping the 'thought' and intention behind the words at all times adds to clear delivery and audibility. Actors use the term 'motivation' for this process. It is very common for the meaning of a phrase to be lost to an audience if the actor has lost concentration on the thought and intention behind the words. Likewise the teacher who does not feel a natural enthusiasm for the subject, or who feels coerced into the teaching of a subject that he or she would rather not teach, can develop audibility problems because they have limited commitment to the words. Actors also learn through experience that at times it is important to allow space between words and phrases in order to allow them to stand out from the others around them, and that intensity of feeling and commitment can aid audibility. Physical stillness and a low intense vocal volume are often used for the most significant of speeches, yet despite the low volume these can still be heard clearly. In addition they are concerned with the energized use of consonants, particularly the final ones that define words. An example of this is the difference between the words 'road', 'rogue', 'roam', 'rose' and 'rope', when spoken. The definition of the last consonant is needed if the word is going to be heard and understood, otherwise confusion can occur when final consonants are ill-defined. Speech is made up of voiced and voiceless sounds. In large spaces it is the voiced sounds that carry, because they set up vibrations in the space.

To experience this, use the spoken voiced /z/ in the place of the spelt /s/ in the following words and notice the difference that the resonance in the voiced sound makes. We do not use these in close conversation but they are necessary in larger spaces or when speaking to larger groups:

eyes	*ears*	*hands*	*faces*
has	*is*	*was*	*his*
hers	*knees*	*ideas*	*calls*
pens	*roads*	*seas*	*easy*

Now try:

> *Friends, Romans, countrymen, lend me your ears;*
> *I come to bury Caesar, not to praise him.*

> Julius Caesar by William Shakespeare (Act 3, scene 2)

All vowels are voiced and can significantly help the carrying power of the voice but in contemporary speech we tend to undervalue the vowels and do not give them their full length or energy. Some people perceive those who commit fully to vowels to be flamboyant and extrovert, personality traits that we shy away from. This is unfortunate because vowels also carry enormous musical and emotional value and if used fully give both resonance and range to the voice, while at the same time increasing carrying power.

Exercise

Take the vowels out of the following words and string them together without the intrusion of any consonants:

> *How sweet the moonlight sleeps upon this bank!*

> Merchant of Venice by William Shakespeare (Act 5, scene 1)

When you find the innate musical and emotional value of the vowels you also tap into the larger vocal resonance of the voice. Notice the way the vowel sounds carry; because they are voiced and continuing, they have vocal 'body'. If we can balance speech with more vowel sounds, we immediately develop a greater ability to fill the space easily. Sometimes this can be achieved by simply slowing down.

In the theatre, what audiences often consider inaudible is in fact perfectly loud. What it lacks, more often than not, is clear intention and definition. These are aspects that teachers can work on and that will improve delivery and therefore audibility immediately. Any teacher working too hard to produce a louder volume is likely to 'lock' breath and neck, thus reducing peripheral vision, raising the pitch and giving an impression of aggression that may lead to a loss of goodwill and attention from the class.

When working with actors it becomes apparent that the loudest volumes (which are not used all that often by actors and certainly not for prolonged periods) are sustainable with very little effort when they come from a free and open body position. The minute the neck locks, high volume is not an option without causing vocal discomfort. The actor works to find ways of producing volume without 'closing down' the open neck position. Above all the actor fills the space physically and vocally without 'pushing' to reach the back. Most actors work to develop an omnidirectional approach, because so many theatres today are not built with a proscenium arch and often there are audience members behind, as well as in front of them. An actor–audience relationship is not unlike that of the modern teacher who, it is said, 'needs eyes in the back of the head'. This omnidirectional approach involves keeping an active level of communication going all the time, developing the peripheral vision, using voice that is resonant and therefore has carrying power, and using defined consonants and receiving as well as emitting energy. In terms of the space itself, it is important to see it being inhabited by the audience as well by the actor or teacher. There should never be an 'us and them' approach, because this is likely to promote a feeling of alienation. Actors usually walk about the space in order to familiarize themselves with it and to find out how their voices behave within the space. Once they have a feel for the natural acoustic of the space, they can modify their voice accordingly.

Exercises

There are specific techniques that often prove successful in gaining a centred physical stillness and a vocal quality that is unrestricted by the neck muscles going into the extreme positions of 'fight' or 'flight/flee'. These exercises work because there is a changed attitude in the speaker who, instead of submitting to the urge to reach out, or (in extreme cases) to 'punch' out to the class with the voice, stands his or her ground and imagines that the voice is beginning at the back of the classroom and travelling towards him or her.

The 'towards strategy'

1. *Moving from the wall:* find a spot on the wall and, standing a few inches from it, concentrate on voicing the sound /mah/ and placing the sound on the spot. Once you have established this keep concentrating on the spot but slowly move backwards away from the wall. You may find at first that you run out of breath quite quickly, but with practice this will improve and you will find that you can move further away without loss of breath. It is important to become aware of the sound being drawn away from the point of concentration and towards yourself. The neck and head never thrust forward and the body remains 'open'. As you continue to do the exercise, increase the arc of sound so that, instead of describing a straight line from the wall to yourself, you allow the sound to arc upwards and over towards you. The arc is used because it explores vocal range and in speech we use vocal range all the time.

2. *Calling:* imagine that you are on a boat or mountain top and that you are calling to a friend on another boat or mountain top. Neither point of focus is at an uncomfortable distance, but you will need to use an extended sound. Place your hands to your mouth and call in a moderate volume, 'Hello there'. The person pretending to be on the second boat or hill answers, also using the call. If improvisation is a problem, a simple question and answer such as 'How are you?', 'Very well, thank you' can be planned beforehand. The call is best seen as a continuous sound that lifts and arcs from the mouth of the caller to the ear of the receiver. Shouting should never be used for the exercise, which is about sustaining sound and can be done, with practice, with very little volume.

3. *Attracting attention:* use the exclamation 'Hey!' in order to attract somebody's attention at the other side of the room. In this exercise it is important to avoid an aggressive approach because in aggressive mode the sound is forced out. The neck and jaw will thrust forward and the habitual laryngeal setting is altered; the larynx is compressed – often accompanied by vocal discomfort. The fists will often clench, and the shoulder girdle will invariably tighten. The knees will generally lock. It is therefore very important to work in a non-aggressive manner.

   Try instead to imagine that the starting point of the sound is from the individual whose attention you want to attract. Instead of pushing the sound out from yourself, draw it towards you. Try using the hands and arms to help you draw the sound slowly over the space until it reaches you. The sound becomes elongated and the vowel is used to allow the sound to travel. This allows you to hold your centred physical position. The head need not be thrust forward; in fact you can retain optimum alignment and the neck can remain free, allowing the peripheral vision to be maintained.

4. *Pickpocket:* using the image of drawing sound towards yourself over the space, imagine that you are lifting a scarf out of the pocket of a passer-by. Start by standing fairly close to her and saying the phrase, 'The scarf is mine' as you move away from the passer-by. Elongate the vowels and lift and arc the voice, as if it travelled with the scarf, from the pocket to you.

4a. The second part of the exercise is to start further away from the passer-by and vocally 'hook' the scarf and some money out of the imagined pocket. Use the phrase, 'The money and scarf are mine'. The use of /m/ aids the voice because it is resonant and a continuous consonant. You should experience a feeling of sustaining sound as you did in the calling exercise.

5. *Fishing exercise:* this is similar to the pickpocket exercise. Imagine a fishing line that you have already cast. Establish where the line and hook have landed and this will become the focal point for your sound. Take in breath easily and without tension and release it on /mah/ as you reel the line in towards yourself. Once the 'drawing towards' of the line has been established, you can develop the exercise by gently increasing volume as the line travels towards you. As with the other exercises the head and neck should not be thrust outward, but stay in a balanced and unfixed position on the spine while voicing.

The principle of all these exercises is that you draw sound towards yourself and from the point of communication, rather than pushing it out towards the point of communication. This is quite obviously an image that goes against physical science; nevertheless it keeps the body aligned and is a great aid in the struggle against the tendency to thrust sound out, locking neck and losing all sense of coordinated speech and communication.

If the habitual use of voice has been quiet, a louder sound might feel overbearing or simply unnatural. It is important to be able to use the voice to achieve your goals and this may mean developing new styles of vocal usage. Rather than 'changing your voice' you should strive to explore a number of options, which might be useful in a number of situations.

If you suspect that your lack of volume is connected to fear of speaking, try the following checklist before you begin.

Volume checklist

The first step is to release the physical tension. A 'checklist' should remind you to:

1. Release shoulders
2. Free neck (occipital joint)
3. Release jaw and tongue
4. Open the chest by grasping the hands behind you and stretching arms upwards.

Once this is achieved:

1. Stand with weight on both feet
2. Look at your audience and see them as friendly, willing and wanting to hear you. Generally speaking the audience wants you to succeed.
3. Shift the anxiety from yourself to them. That means you want them to have your knowledge or share your experience.
4. Avoid breath-holding. Breathe out and then allow new air to enter the body just before you begin.
5. Smile before you start speaking.

This may all seem impossible to begin with but it gets easier. At the same time you need technically to develop vocal muscle, freedom and resonance.

Playful exercises for volume

Having done the breathing exercises in Chapter 11, it is important to release sound freely. These exercises require a sense of humour because if you feel self-conscious you will hold on to the sound rather than release it.

1. Using the sound /YAH/ /YAH/ /YAH/ let your jaw be loose and free. Allow yourself to look 'gormless' and ridiculous.

2. Blow a raspberry /BRRRR/ or /PRRRR/ through the lips. This engages and harnesses the breath and you can feel its effects on the lips.

3. Working in pairs, imagine that you are playing tennis. Using an imagined racquet and the sound /doh/ as a ball (any sound beginning with B or D will work), hit the sound very firmly over the 'net' making sure that it reaches your partner. As you get better at sustaining the sound through the air, try lifting and curving the sound.

4. Feel that your weight is centred in the hips and pelvis – imagine that you are dragging yourself through mud. Speak as you do this. *Three Blind Mice* will do!

5. Sitting on a chair bounce yourself up and down and bounce the sound out as you speak. Try to shake yourself like a 'jelly' while letting out the sound /ooo/ /ahh/.

6. Lean up against a wall and rhythmically bounce your back against the wall while drunkenly speaking *Three Blind Mice* – allow the sound to release with each impact.

7. Feel the vibrations in your chest as you sound /MAH/. Beat the chest with the fist of one or both hands and allow the sound to release with the impact.

8. Laugh with a mock 'Santa Clause' laugh using HO! HO! HO! Do not be concerned if the sound is not genuine. Turn the HO! into an elongated call across a distance, lifting and dropping the sound as it travels through the air.

9. Turn the distance call into a phrase such as Over here! This way! Ahoy there! etc.

Placement exercises

You will not be able to create volume if the voice is trapped at the back of the mouth. Placing the voice in the mask of the face is best for the production of volume. Test your placement by placing your fingers over your nose and speaking this exercise:

/b/ /b/ /b/ /bah/

/g/ /g/ /g/ /gah/

The sound should be completely forward and free and should not enter the nose at all. If it does, it indicates tension in the tongue, soft palate or back of the throat.

Now speak a phrase. It is important to choose a phrase that does not contain the nasal sounds /m/ /n/ /ng/; the following are useful:

This is the house that Jack built.

Workers built the old wall by the field.

The path through the woods is used by walkers.

How sorry he was to see her go.

You will notice that in order to produce the clear sound you need to free the jaw and increase the space in the mouth, use more breath support and 'think' the voice forward and on to the lips. These actions all increase the volume and forward projection of the voice.

Volume exercises using verse

1. Speak the first line on a quiet volume.

2. The next should be louder.

3. The following louder still.

4. Continue until you are as loud as you can comfortably be.

5. Keep the neck, head and shoulders free.

6. Keep the attitude playful and relaxed. Avoid trying too hard.

7. Do not shout or lose support.

When you are happy that you have mastered this exercise, reverse the order, starting loudly and getting quieter.

You can do these exercises walking away and/or toward the wall, increasing volume as you leave the wall and decreasing it as you return to it. Then:

1. Sing a line quietly/speak it quietly with the same support.

2. Sing/speak it with more volume and sustained support.

3. Continue to sing and speak more and more loudly.

Make sure that you add range as you add volume. To explore range, imagine that you are sweeping the voice from the floor to the ceiling. Use all the range at your disposal. Notice how this frees the volume. Then:

1. Count from one to ten getting louder all the time.

2. Repeat the counting exercise very slowly.

3. Repeat once more, making sure that you extend the vowels in each word. Vowels are voiced and carry both resonance and volume. Do not worry about the strange quality that this produces. The balance between vowel and consonant can be redressed later.

4. Try speaking a typical classroom phrase, increasing volume each time you speak.

5. Sing the phrase, noticing the increased volume, and then speak it once more attempting the same volume.

If the sound is not free, tap the chest or jump up and down to release the sound. Alternatively, sitting on the floor or a chair bounce, jog or shake the sound out of the body.

It is important to remember that too much effort will block volume rather than create it. Being able to play is an important attribute if volume is the goal.

Although it is important to be able to create volume, it can be a strategy that is over-used. Volume as a norm can be as monotonous as sustained quiet speech. Variety that is responsive and appropriate to the subject matter and situation is ideal. At times it is necessary to look at the alternatives, especially if the voice is suffering.

This observation comes from a trainee teacher, Kate Herbert (2003, p. 6), who wrote a diary detailing her experience:

> I have a sore throat. A large night out with fellow trainees and another snowy commute on the scooter resulted in a weekend in bed and no voice to speak of in the classroom come Monday. It works! Apparently all trainees believe that a raised voice works. This week's muffled squeaks have produced improved sound effects from the children – near silence. Teaching evaporation in science and stencils in art has worked better for my lack of vocal chords [sic] than anything previously. We continue to learn something new every day.

Trying to produce volume on an ailing voice, whatever the reason for the malaise, is not advisable.

Healthy shouting

We know that it is possible to shout without hurting or damaging the voice. Nevertheless many teachers trace a vocal problem back to an incident when they, frustrated and angry, have shouted at a child or group of children. They feel a catch in the throat, a loss of vocal freedom and experience a need to force the sound out. They feel the result immediately as roughness in the larynx, a hoarse raspy sound or reduced range. They then proceed to attempt to clear the throat but generally to no avail.

Children in the playground, however, seem able to shout, call, yell and even shriek with no problems. They are being playful and therefore they are free of tension. There is often a quality of laughter lurking beneath the shout. If you look at their faces you see the open expression, which is also mirrored by the body posture. The head is aligned, the chest open. The sense of fun removes the tension in the upper body, and generally children are running when they shout and the release that this action gives to the voice avoids the chance of damage. There are exceptions and some children have to be taught to shout without harming the voice. Actors, too, are often able to produce blood-curdling cries and yells without damage. It must be said that many of them have to work at it, to find a technique that works against the emotion of the moment.

All the calling and 'toward' exercises in this section are important for the development of a healthy 'shout' but here is a work-out designed to assist the process. It is important to warm up the voice before attempting the shouting exercises and to precede them with breathing exercises and exercises that release tension in the pharynx and the area of the larynx. If you begin to experience discomfort, it is a signal to stop the exercises and return to breath support work. It is also vital to have a clear idea of your point of focus, i.e. of the individual or groups with whom you wish to communicate. Although the term 'shouting' conjures up ideas of anger, it is always inadvisable to use high volume if you are angry. When you are angry it is very difficult to separate energy and tension, and often 'inexperienced' shouters are not able to use high energy without constriction, especially if they have to deal with the additional stresses involved in feelings of anger. It is much more effective to use a controlled and supported sound because any indication of anger suggests a loss of control on the part of the speaker and this undermines authority, rather than increasing it. By removing focus from the larynx and using breath support effectively, you can successfully produce a very high volume without hurting the voice. There are other helpful strategies, such as increasing the precision of the articulation and using greater vocal range than normal, that remove the need to resort to excessive volume.

Shouting work-out

1. It is important to precede this with work on shoulder, neck and jaw release. It is not recommended that you begin work on shouting until you have developed an awareness of tension that may exist in the jaw and have been able to minimize it.

2. Do the second exercise under 'Breathing exercises' of Chapter 11. This involves lying on your stomach with a weight on the buttocks and breathing down as low in the body as possible. Develop the exercise by imagining that the breath leaves the body via each of the vertebrae until it reaches the mouth. Practise this using the voiceless /fff/ and then use a gentle /mmm/. Once you have established the journey of the /mmm/, begin it in the coccyx and increase the energy as you travel up the spine; when you approach the shoulder blades open the sound into a vowel, e.g. /mmmah/. Repeat the exercise using different vowels such as /mmmaw/, /mmmoh/, /mmmoo/. Allow the voice to change pitch and to lift and arc as you release the sound. As long as you 'begin' the sound well below the level of the larynx, it is possible to develop considerable volume without restriction.

3. *The yoga cat*: kneel on all fours, and keep your hands directly below the shoulders. As you breathe in, curve the lower back up towards the ceiling as the head tucks in towards the chest. As you breathe out, allow the lower back to sink towards the floor as you imagine the breath moving up through the spine and, as the head comes up and eyes look towards the ceiling, allow the breath to leave the body.

4. After having done this exercise several times on the floor, stand up and vocalize the sound /mmmmmm/ and imagine it travelling up the spine. As it reaches the shoulder blades, open the sound out into an /ah/. It may be easier to start in a bent-over position and to unfold through the spine as you produce the sound, synchronizing the movement with the sound.

   A word of caution: as you release the vowel and lift the eyes upwards do not extend the neck so that you restrict the pharynx.

5. Keep working on this exercise and open to a variety of vowels, e.g. /mmmmm-maw/, /mmmmmmoh/, /mmmmmmay/.

6. Once you are happy with this begin to build volume, feeling the real release of the vowel. Once again never be tempted to start the sound at the level of the larynx. The secret of 'shouting' is to begin the sound well below the level of the throat. By picturing the sound starting in the coccyx you remove the focus and stress from the throat. This is of course an image, but it helps to keep the sound free. At this stage never get louder than is comfortable and keep the exercises in the style of a call.

7. (In pairs) Imagine each of you is on the top of a hill, some distance apart.

Partner A cups their hands around the mouth and calls to B, ' Red roses, who will buy?' B responds, 'How much for a dozen?'

When this is well established and tension free, use the follow lines:

A: *Ill met by moonlight, proud Titania!*

B: *What, jealous Oberon?*

Midsummer Night's Dream by William Shakespeare (Act 2, scene 1)

8. Begin to introduce an attitude of censorship into the dialogue, still keeping the quality of breath support and vocal freedom.

9. Now try some of the phrases that you are likely to use in the teaching situation, e.g. 'Class four, books away, please' or 'Close your desks and stand in line please'. Intone the phrase first on one note, then use the hill-calling exercise and, third, imagine calling it to the group or child in question.

Suggestions for muscularity

Additional muscularity not only increases clarity and volume but also connects words with their inherent meaning and power. An excellent and enriching way of exercising the muscles of speech is to work on extant material. Tongue twisters are useful and can be fun, but can be ill-advised if they are merely 'rattled off' without being related to meaning. There is much wonderfully structured and honed verse available that offers not just a muscular exercise, but stimulation of the imagination and, in addition, demands commitment to rhythm and phrasing. The benefits of using verse are numerous because these passages increase vocabulary, stimulate ideas and discussion, and offer the experience of speaking out loud and exploring the power of language. Verse also has marked rhythm, which connects the speaker with the syllabic energy of language and the ways in which this energy and the heightened language affect the speaker and the audience. As well as verse it is useful to work on well-structured prose and political speeches. These exercise the speaker's ability to share stories and, in the case of political speeches, to persuade and explore the power of words. They are also a useful aid in history classes.

Syllables, stress and clarity in the classroom

Many contemporary speakers pay little attention to the value of the syllables of words. Modern speech is often elided or contracted in an effort

to make it sound friendly or relaxed. Equally, haste can be the cause o
not giving syllables their appropriate value. Many people feel, often cor
rectly, that they are being over-aggressive or pedantic if they give ful
value to syllables. This problem is avoided by not over-stressing and usin
both the stressed and the unstressed syllables in words.

Over-stressing means stressing every word and not observing th
unstressed syllable, and it is this that sounds pedantic and monotonou
because it removes the music from the language. Enjoyment of the musi
cality of words gives them clarity and muscular energy, which is bound u
with defining the syllables and committing to the consonants. As well a
defining the syllable, it is important to release the rhythm by stressing th
appropriate syllable.

First language speakers assimilate the correct stress pattern in words i
their native tongue, but speakers of English as a second language ofter
find this aspect of the language difficult and frustrating because there ar
no concrete rules. One of the most frequent problems in audibility for sec
ond language English speakers is incorrect syllabic stress. Notice hov
changing the stress in the word 'allow' (from unstress/stress t
stress/unstress) makes the word difficult to recognize. An appreciation o
syllables is particularly important in teaching, because it is in the class
room that students are often introduced to a word for the first time
Clearly enunciating syllables not only assists audibility but also helps stu
dents with their spelling.

As well as knowing where the stress falls, it is important to enjoy th
contact with the consonants rather than to smooth over and minimiz
them. Consider the number of syllables in these words:

Library

February

Procrastination

Vulnerable

Multiplication

Eradicate

Giving value to the syllables is a simple and effective way of increasin
audibility. Although elision or contraction is usually acceptable in con
versational speech, once there is distance to cover and information t
exchange, success is more likely if the syllables are given their natura
weight.

The muscular engagement required enhances the articulation of th
word as well as releasing the rhythm and impetus. This avoids monotony

which often results from a lack of syllabic energy and monotonous speech can be difficult to understand.

Problems encountered by second language speakers

Learning the vocabulary and grammar of a language is far easier than learning the stress pattern. In English the stress is often, but not always, on the second syllable (as in the iambic metre), e.g. today, console, society, enjoy, repeat, etc., but may be on the first in words such as exquisite, vulnerable, over, Monday, fifty. When a native speaker hears a word being incorrectly stressed, the meaning is often lost or they take longer to decode and understand it.

Speakers who are rushing will invariably compromise the syllabic value of words as will those who 'shy away' from the physical and mental commitment to the word. This may be because they do not wish to appear forceful or encroach on the personal space of the listener, or because they are over-familiar with the material. Easy confident muscular engagement with syllables gives the audience a sense that the speaker 'owns' the space as well as the subject matter.

A word of caution

Avoid stressing the 'weak' or unstressed syllables because this results in a staccato sound that is as monotonous as not articulating or stressing the appropriate syllables. It may also be perceived as being over-bearing and aggressive. It is important to balance syllabic value with the music and rhythm of the language.

The unstressed neutral vowel

Naturally rhythmical speakers instinctively know when not to stress a syllable. Once again second language speakers may find themselves encountering difficulties and tending to stress too many. The English language is one of 'stress and *unstress*' and the neutral vowel is a great aid to easy rhythm. The sound (not the spelling) of the neutral is 'a' (as in above) and may be found in words such as father, mother, sister, brother, anger, folder, etc. and at the beginning of the following words: abundant, ago. The sound can be spelt in many ways, such as '*er*' in moth*er*, '*a*' in *a*llow.

The /a/ vowel in a phrase such as: *a* book/ *a* pen and a pencil/ *a* cup of tea/ *a* walk in *a* park/ all use the neutral /a/ and should not be sounded /ay book/ ay pen/, etc. Notice how the use of this unstressed vowel allows the rhythm to emerge.

The same applies to the neutral version of /the*e*/. 'The' only becomes /the*e*/ when it precedes a vowel as in the following examples, /the*e* egg/, /the*e* ostrich/, /the*e* inkpot/. Both first and second language speakers will often 'over-correct' this sound and over-stress in an attempt to sound clear and well spoken. Natural sounding speech with flow and rhythm should always be the goal. Second language speakers often find English confusing because it has only five written vowels but these have many sounds, approximately 24 in all, depending on accent and dialect.

Consonants

The connection that consonants have with meaning has been discussed in Chapter 6. Their function as a means of assisting audibility over distance is quite specific. Over half the consonants are voiced, e.g. /b/ is voiced, whereas /p/ is created only with breath, /d/is voiced and /t/ is created only with breath. Examples of other voiced sounds are /m/ /ng/ /n/ /l/ /r/ /z/. As voiced sounds these consonants create vibration and resonance and so enhance audibility. If a speaker engages with the consonant, he or she commits to it in terms of breath and muscle and this too develops the volume. By committing to the word, there is a greater muscularity in the mask of the face and the voice is placed forward and is, therefore, again more audible. There is also a perception of status and confidence produced by firm, committed consonants and the resonance that they produce which, along with easier lip-reading from the audience or class, enhances the speaker's chances of being heard. When speech has lost its spontaneity and become automatic, or when the speaker is not committed to the content of the language or the desire to communicate it, elision of consonant clusters and de-voicing of voiced sounds are much more likely to occur. What then results is dull and inaudible.

Exercises for consonants

These exercises can be done with classes of any age. Try them after the exercises for the articulators described in Chapter 11 in order to get as much benefit as possible.

1. Try to explore the dynamic in the initial consonant of the following words beginning with the consonant /b/. Notice how the breath gathers behind the muscles in the mask of the face, behind the lips. Build up the pressure before exploding the sound through on the following words, using as much physical movement and energy as you can: *burst/bubble/bounce/bound*.

2. In the same way explore the dynamic of /d/ when saying the following words: *dash/direct/destroy/daub/*.

3. Explore the dynamic of /g/ when saying the following words: *giggle/gash/grapple/gush/*.

4. Explore the dynamic of /n/ when saying the following words: *niggle/nuzzle/nimble/nudge/*.

5. Explore the dynamic of /z/ in different positions within the words when saying: *zoom/ooze/lazy/fizz/*.

6. Imagine that you are playing tennis and 'bat' consonants over the net with energy, using good breath support and experiencing the build up and release of the breath on the initial consonant.

7. Once you have done that, create a 'tennis match', using two people to serve and return words, which begin with plosive consonants, exploring light and flexible sound and movement as well as the forceful dynamic, e.g.

ball/bash/bounce

diver/delve/dash

gird/glide/glimmer

move/murmur/mumble

lash/lob/limp

8. Work on difficult consonant combinations to exercise and make demands on the flexibility and agility of the articulators. Here are some examples:

sixth form (which is often reduced to sick form)

fifth (which becomes fif)

text (which becomes tex)

precinct (which becomes precing)

subject (which becomes subjec)

Conclusion

The context in which the exercises and strategies outlined in this book will be applied will be different for each individual, depending on the specific vocal demands that he or she encounters. The essential work undertaken by those who choose to teach is reliant on a flexible and free vocal mechanism, and on the teacher's ability to convert thoughts and ideas into sounds, words and language. The fact that we take our voices so much for granted and think about them only when they do not work effectively is an indication of the general resilience of the voice and the synchronicity of thought and speech. When a problem does occur, it is often as a result of an increase in tension or stress, which alters the fine balance that usually exists between the production of voice and the effort levels required to achieve easy and effortless voicing.

The successful school answers the needs of both the students and staff. Raising the awareness of vocal needs among teachers, head teachers, governors, and those in charge of the education authorities and educational training colleges is therefore of paramount importance.

Voice problems can be successfully treated by specialists in the field of voice and it is important not to sacrifice a career that you love because of lack of specialist intervention. The help is out there. Go and get it.

This book will have been productive if, through its cocktail of early warning signs, anatomical information, strategies and exercises, it raises awareness of voice in general, promotes good vocal hygiene, and helps to steer teachers and professional voice users who are experiencing difficulty towards the help that they need and can so easily find.

In industry and commerce the focus is now on investment in staff in order to increase productivity; the focus in education must be on the teachers who deliver it. Many teachers who want to remain within the profession are unable to withstand the high levels of stress, stress that is often manifested in a voice problem, and move to less stressful careers.

It is our hope that this book may provide the necessary support, information and guidance to halt this inexorable process.

Appendix: useful contacts

British Performing Arts Medicine Trust
18 Ogle Street, London W1P 7LG
Website: www.bpamt.co.uk

The British Voice Association
Institute of Laryngology and Otology, 330 Gray's Inn Road, London WC1X 8EE
Website: www.british-voice-association.com

The British Wheel of Yoga
25 Jermyn Street, Sleaford, Lincs NG34 7RU
Website: www.bwy.org.uk or www.yogauk.com

The English Speaking Union
Dartmouth House, 37 Charles Street, London WC1
Website: www.esu.org

The International Centre for Voice
Central School of Speech and Drama, Eton Avenue, London NW3 3HY
Email: voice@cssd.ac.uk

The Royal College of Speech and Language Therapists
2 White Hart Yard, London SE1 1NX
Website: www.rcslt.org

Society of Teachers of the Alexander Technique
20 London House, 266 Fulham Road, London SW10 9EL
Website: www.stat.org.uk

The Society of Teachers of Speech and Drama
The Secretary, 73 Berry Hill Road, Mansfield, Notts NG18 4RU
Website: www.stad.org.uk

Voice Care Network
Co-ordinator: Roz Comins, 29 Southbank Road, Kenilworth, Warwicks CV8 1LA
Website: www.voicecare.org.uk

Warwickshire Education Development Service
Advisory Service, Manor Hall, Sandy Lane, Lemington Spa, Warwicks CV32 6RD
Website: www.warwickshire.gov.uk

Theatre education departments

Royal Shakespeare Company
Education Department, Waterside, Stratford-upon-Avon, Warks CV36 6BB
Website: www.rsc.org.uk

The National Theatre
Education Department, Upper Ground, South Bank, London SE1 9PX
Website: www.nt-online.org.uk

Globe Theatre
21 New Globe Walk, Bankside, London SE1 9DT
Website: www.shakespeares-globe.org

The English National Opera
Education Department, St Martins Lane, London WC2N 4ES
Website: www.eno.org.uk

BBC Education Information Unit
White City, London W12 7TS
Website: www.bbc.co.uk

Other useful websites

Seal (Society for Effective/Affective Learning)
Website: www.seal.org.uk

The Feldenkrais Guild UK
Website: www.feldenkrais.co.uk

Teacher Support Network
Website: www.teachernet.gov.uk

References

Aaltonen T (1989) A comparison of subjective voice complaints of teachers in Northern and Southern Finland. A Licentiate thesis University of Oulu, Department of Logopedics and Phonetics Oulu

Aronsen AE (1985) Clinical Voice Disorders. New York: Thième-Stratton

Atkinson M (1984) Our Masters' Voices. London: Routledge

Berliner W (2003) Paperwork overload. The Guardian 13/5/2003

Berry C (1992) Shakespeare Comes to Broadmoor. In Cox M (ed.), That Secret Voice. London: Jessica Kingsley

Berry C (1993) The Actor and the Text. London: Virgin

Blunkett D (1998) Speech to AoC annual conference, reported in FEDA Editorial. Reform, 1999, 2

Borrild K (1978) Classroom acoustics. In: Ross M, Giolos TG (eds), Auditory Management of Hearing-Impaired Children. Baltimore: University Park Press

Brodnitz FS (1965) Vocal Rehabilitation, 5th edn. Rochester, MN: American Academy of Ophthalmology and Otolaryngology

Brown GA (1980) Explaining: studies from the higher education context. Final report to SRRC. University of Nottingham

Brown GA (1986) Explaining. In: Hargie O (ed.), A Handbook of Communication Skills. London: Croom Helm

Bufton E (1997) An investigation in to the changes occurring between 1992 and 1997 in the number of teachers presenting with voice disorders at selected voice clinics in the United Kingdom: the provision of voice care education for trainee teachers. Unpublished BSc (Hons) project, Central School of Speech and Drama, London

Cains R (1995) The perceptions, experiences and needs of newly qualified teachers – a longitudinal study. Unpublished PhD thesis, University of Hull

Carvel J (2000) Constant carping upsets teachers. The Guardian 3/1/00

Chan RWC (1994) Does the voice improve with vocal hygiene? A study of some instrumental voice measures in a group of kindergarten teachers. Journal of Voice 8: 279–91

Charter D (2000) Pay for trainees doubles interest in teaching. The Times 19/5/02

Clowry P (1996) Letter. The Times 30/12/96

Coates TJ, Thoresen CE (1976) Teacher anxiety: a review with recommendations. Review of Educational Research 46: 159–84

Comins R (1995) A pilot study of classroom noise levels and teachers' reactions. Voice 4: 127–34

Cooper CL (1968) Job distress: recent research and the emerging role of the clinical psychologist. Bulletin of British Psychological Society 339: 325–31

Cooper M (1973) Modern Techniques of Vocal Rehabilitation, 2nd edn. Springfield, IL: Charles C Thomas

Coopers and Lybrand Deloitte (1994) Cost of the National Curriculum in primary schools: commissioned by the National Union of Teachers. In: Evans L, Packwood A, Neill SRStJ, Campbell RJ (eds), The Meaning of Infant Teachers' Work. London: Routledge

Council Directive (1989) On the introduction of measures to encourage improvements in the safety and health of workers at work. 89/391/EEC Brussels

Department for Education (1992) Circular No. 9/92 (25/6/92)

DfES (2001) Healthy Schools, Healthy Teachers website: www.dfes.gov.uk/hsht

DfES (2003) Raising standards and tackling work-load: a national agreement. January 2003

Dragone MLS, Reos R, Sichirolli S, Behlau M (1998) A longitudinal analysis of the teaching voice. Proceedings 24th Congress of International Association of Logopedics and Phoniatrics. Amsterdam: Numegen University Press

Dunham J (1983) Coping with stress in schools. Special Education: Forward Trends 106(2): 6–9

Dunkin MJ, Biddle BJ (1974) The Study of Teaching. New York: Holt, Rinehart & Winston.

Edwards AD, Furlong VJ (1978) The Language of Teaching. London: Heinemann

Evans l, Packwood A, Neill SRStJ, Campbell RJ (eds) (1994) The Meaning of Infant Teachers' Work. London: Routledge

Farb P (1973) Word Play. London: Cape

Further Education National Training Organisation (FENTO) (1999) Standards Framework Consultation Document. London: FENTO

Hargreaves A (1984) The significance of classroom coping strategies. In: Hargreaves A, Woods P (eds), Classrooms and Staffrooms. Milton Keynes: Open University Press

Hart W (1934) Teachers and Teaching. London: Macmillan

Health and Safety Commission Schools Education Advisory Committee (SEAC) (2003) Voice Matters, Summer, No. 29

Herbert K (2003) Diary of a trainee teacher. The Guardian 11/2/03

Herrington-Hall K, Lee L, Stemple J, Niemi K, Miller-McHone M (1998) Description of laryngeal pathologies by age, sex and occupation in a treatment seeking sample. Journal of Speech and Hearing Disorder 53: 57–64

Hirano M, Kurita S, Nakashima T (1983) Growth, development and ageing of human vocal folds. In: Blass DM, Abbs JH (eds), Vocal Fold Physiology. San Diego: College Hill Press

Honey J (1989) Does Accent Matter? London: Faber & Faber

Hunt J, Slater A (2003) Working with Children's Voice Disorders. Bicester: Speechmark

Jackson PW (1968) Life in Classrooms. New York: Holt, Rinehart & Winston

Jones NS, Lannigan FJ, McMullagh M, Anggiansah A, Owen W, Harris TM (1990) Acid reflux and hoarseness. Journal of Voice 4: 355–8

Koufman JA (1998) What are voice disorders and who gets them? Website: www.bgsm.edu/voice/voice_disorders.html

Lass NJ, Ruscello DM, Stout LL, Hoffman FM (1991) Peer perceptions of normal and voice disordered children. Folio Phoniatrica Logopedics 43, 29–35

Lightfoot E (1999) Teachers get free stress helpline. The Daily Telegraph 9/9/99

Macdonald G (1994) The Alexander Technique. London: Hodder

Martin S (1994) Voice care and development for teachers: survey report. Voice 3: 32–43

Martin S (2003) An exploration of factors which have an impact on the vocal performance and vocal effectiveness of newly qualified teachers/lecturers. Unpublished PhD thesis, University of Greenwich

Martin S, Darnley L (1996) The Teaching Voice. London: Whurr Publishers

Masuda T, Ikeda Y, Manako H, Komiyana S (1993) Analysis of vocal abuse: fluctuations in phonation time and intensity in four groups of speakers. Acta Otolaryngologica 113: 547–52

Mathieson L (2001) Greene and Mathieson's The Voice and its Disorders, 6th edn. London: Whurr Publishers

Mehrabian A (1972) Nonverbal Communication. Chicago: Aldine

Mersbergen MR van, Verdolini K, Titze IR (1999) Fatigue effects on the voice. Journal of Voice 13: 518–28

Milne S (1999) Job insecurity leads to stress epidemic. The Guardian 5/1/99

Morton V, Watson DR (1998) The teaching voice: problems and perceptions. Logopedics Phoniatrics Vocology 23: 133–9

Morton V, Watson DR (1999) Dysphonia in the classroom: a double-edged sword. Presented at IIIrd Pan European Voice Conference, Utrecht, The Netherlands

Moses PJ (1954) The Voice of Neurosis. New York: Grune & Stratton

Ogunleye J (2002) An investigation of curriculum arrangements conducive to fostering creativity in post-compulsory education and training institutions. Unpublished PHD thesis, University of Greenwich, London

Ohlsson AC (1993) Preventative voice care for teachers. Voice 2: 112–15

Owen G (2002) A fifth of teachers moonlight to make ends meet. The Times 20/5/2002

Pekkarinen E, Viljanen V (1991) Acoustic conditions for speech communication in classrooms. Scandinavica Audiologica 20: 257–63

Powell T (1997) Free Yourself from Harmful Stress. London: Dorling Kindersley

Ramig LO, Verdolini K (1998) Treatment efficacy: voice disorders. Journal of Speech and Language Hearing Research 41: S101–16

Rogers C (1975) A Way of Being. Boston: Houghton Mifflin

Sapir S, Attias J, Sharar A (1992) Vocal attrition related to idiosyncratic dysphonia: re-analysis of survey data. European Journal of Disorders of Communication 27(2): 1

Sapir S, Keidar A, Mathers-Schmidt B (1993) Vocal attrition in teachers: survey findings. European Journal of Disorders of Communication 28: 177–85

Smithers R (1999) Actors may train teachers' voices. The Guardian 29/7/99

Smithers A, Robinson P (2003) Teachers leaving. Cited in Berliner (2003)

Smythe RL, Bamford JM (1997) Speech perception of hearing impaired children in mainstream acoustic environments: an exploratory study. Deafness and Education (JBATOD) 21(2): 26–31

The Stationery Office (1997) Guidelines for Environmental Design in Schools (revision of Design Note 17). Building Bulletin 87

Teacher Training Agency (2002) Qualifying to Teach. PubTPU 0803/02-02

Titze IR, Lemke J, Montequin D (1997) Populations in the US workforce who rely on voice as a primary tool of trade: a preliminary report. Journal of Voice 11: 254–9

Travers CJ, Cooper CL (1993) Mental Health, job satisfaction and occupational stress among UK teachers. Journal of Occupation and Stress 7: 203–19

Travers CJ, Cooper CL (1996).Teachers under Pressure. London: Routledge

Verdolini-Marston K, Sandage M, Titze IR (1994) Effect of hydration treatments on laryngeal nodules and polyps and related voice measures. Journal of Voice 8: 30–47

Vilkman E (2001) A survey on the occupational safety and health arrangements for voice and speech professionals in Europe. In: Dejonckere P (ed.), Occupational Voice: Care and cure. The Hague: Kugler Publications

The Voice Care Network, UK (1996) Voice Matters – The newsletter of Voice Care Network UK, June: p. 4

Ward L (2003) Mocking can scar children. The Guardian 28/10/03

West R, Ansberry M, Carr A (1957) The Rehabilitation of Speech. New York: Harper

Wragg EC (1973) A study of student teachers in the classroom. In: Chanan G (ed.), Towards a Science of Teaching. Slough: NFER

Wu J (1998) School work environment and its impact on the professional competence of newly qualified teachers. Journal of In-Service Education 24(2): 213–25

Index